THE

# Change
# Your
# Biology
# Diet

# THE Change Your Biology Diet

THE PROVEN PROGRAM FOR
LIFELONG WEIGHT LOSS

## Louis J. Aronne, M.D.
### with Diane Reverand

HOUGHTON MIFFLIN HARCOURT
BOSTON • NEW YORK
2016

This book presents the research, experiences, and ideas of its author. It is not intended to be a substitute for consultation with a professional healthcare provider. Consult with your healthcare provider before starting any diet. The publisher and the author disclaim responsibility for any adverse effects resulting directly from information contained in this book.

For information about permission to reproduce selections from this book, write to trade.permissions@hmhco.com or to Permissions, Houghton Mifflin Harcourt Publishing Company, 3 Park Avenue, 19th Floor, New York, New York 10016.

www.hmhco.com

*Library of Congress Cataloging-in-Publication Data is available.*
ISBN 978-0-544-53575-6

Design by Alex Camlin
Illustrations by Josh McKible
Diagrams by Mapping Specialists

Printed in the United States of America
DOC 10 9 8 7 6 5 4 3 2 1

*To our patients whose illness, frustration, and tears have inspired us to develop new ideas and more effective treatments. We believe you.*

# Contents

Foreword ........................................................................ ix

**AUTHOR'S NOTE**
The #1 Health Care Problem ................................... xi

**INTRODUCTION**
Have You Ever Noticed that Your Weight Goes Up,
But Won't Go Down? ................................................ xvii

**PART 1** *It's Not Your Fault*

1  A Plan that Works ................................................. 3
2  Fattening Factors ................................................. 27
3  Why Don't People Just Lose Weight? ................. 56

**PART 2** *The Change Your Biology Program*

4  Winning the Hunger Games .............................. 79
5  The Breakthrough Dozen: 12 Proven Strategies
   for Lifelong Weight Control ............................... 102
6  The Quick Start Change Your Biology Diet ........ 114
7  The Change Your Biology Diet ........................... 135
8  14 Days of Change Your Biology Diet
   Meal Plans ......................................................... 152
9  Quick, Easy, and Delicious Recipes ................... 163
10  Stand Up and Start Moving ............................ 211

**PART 3** *Beyond Diet & Exercise*

11  Medications: A New Frontier ......................... 249
12  The Surgical Solution for Severe Obesity ....... 263

Afterword ................................................................ 285
Acknowledgments .................................................. 289
Selected Sources .................................................... 291
About The Author .................................................. 312
Index ....................................................................... 313
Recipe Index ........................................................... 326

# FOREWORD

DR. LOU ARONNE has been my friend for thirty years. As a young man I was attracted to Lou, because he looked nice in a lab coat. A few years later, he saved me from a massive heart attack, forcing me to take a treadmill stress test—we discovered all of my arteries had turned to cement. Lou believes it was too many potato chips.

A year later, I had quintuple bypass heart surgery. In the middle of the operation the anesthesiologist brought me around and asked if I would like to hold my own heart. Of course this didn't happen. I think it's illegal! But what if it had? Boy, that would be a book. If it wasn't for Lou, I'd be dead, or certainly not in the top physical condition of my life. Which, if any of you have seen me lately, would be difficult to dispute.

Lou has devoted his life to helping the world understand food, obesity, and how to win BIG playing online poker! Lou has a wonderful wife named Jane—in her own right, a championship tennis player. Lou and Jane have two lovely grown children, whose names I can never remember.

This book will help you feel better, lose weight, and make you as smart as Alex Trebek.

Thanks to Lou I understand the connection between heart disease and blood sugar. For me it's an on going project—and my only project since retiring from show business. (I used to be on television.)

Let Lou help how you think and eat. He might save your life as well.

*Dave Letterman*

# The #1 Health Care Problem

WHY DON'T PEOPLE JUST LOSE WEIGHT? If losing weight were easy, two-thirds of adults in this country would not have weight problems. All it would take is cutting calories. It's more complicated than a matter of willpower. Obviously, something else is going on that makes weight management so difficult.

When I lecture new students at Weill Cornell Medical College, I explain the limits of willpower in weight loss with a simple demonstration. I ask a student to hold her breath for a few seconds, then for longer and longer intervals. I instruct the student to do this every day and to hold her breath for five more seconds every week. In a year, she should be able to hold her breath for an hour, right? At that point, everyone in the class laughs at the ridiculous notion. They know their classmate's body won't allow her to hold her breath that long. Something tells her to breathe, because she's suffocating. Strong physical signals will communicate to her that her brain is starved for oxygen. The same thing happens with weight control. Something signals you to eat, because you're starving. It's not as immediate as breathing. Instead of reaching a crisis point in a matter of minutes, it might take days or weeks with eating, but it's the exact same mechanism.

If I do anything in writing this book, my primary goal is to reassure you that having difficulty losing weight is a medical problem, not a lack of self-control. When you try to lose weight or hit a plateau on a diet, do you get the sense that you are struggling against something? In fact, you are. I call it weight loss resistance. Research has given us new insight into what is behind weight gain and how your body resists losing weight. We have discovered that eating too much highly processed, starchy, sweet, fatty food damages the appetite-control center in your brain and precipitates other changes in your body that contribute to fat production and storage. I want to share what we now know about breaking through the physical barriers to weight loss. With a greater understanding of how the body controls weight, we have been able to create diets that work better than ever. What does "work better" mean? It means that it's easier to stick with the plan and that you can lose as much weight as possible. *The Change Your Biology Diet* offers you a science-based program and a set of strategies to help you alter the biological processes that are preventing you from losing weight and keeping it off.

How I came to specialize in obesity and weight management is a classic story of finding a calling. When I was a Fellow in Internal Medicine at Weill Cornell, funded by the Kaiser Foundation, in the mid-eighties, I became interested in cost-effective care — in other words, the economics of health care. Increasingly sophisticated technology had made intensive care units an important part of hospital treatment by the mid-seventies. I set out to do a cost analysis of who should go into intensive care. I was intrigued to discover that patients who were obese cost two or three times more to care for than patients of average weight.

At the same time I was performing this study, I had a patient at the clinic in her late thirties, who needed a walker to get around. Her coronary arteries were severely diseased. She was about five feet two or three and weighed 250 pounds. I wondered how someone so young could be so sick and what we could do to help her. Being that overweight was not as common then as it is today. It seemed obvious that losing weight would be a good start. I found myself thinking about how we could solve her weight problem and whether losing weight would restore her health. At that time, there was no proven relationship between obesity and illness. We could not explain what fat cells had to do with overall health.

When I joined the faculty of New York Hospital-Cornell Medical Center in 1986 along with two other doctors, the chairman wanted each of us to set up a program. Dr. Orli Etingin, one new faculty member, worked on building the Woman's Health Center; Dr. Jonathan Jacobs, the other, set up the Center for Special Studies, which focused on HIV. When I suggested an obesity program, the chairman, Dr. R. Gordon Douglas, had the foresight to think it was a good idea. At the time, being overweight was considered strictly a behavioral problem, but we suspected there was a lot more to the story. If it were simply a matter of cutting calories, overweight people would not have such a struggle dropping excess pounds. We were one of the first research and treatment programs in the country devoted to helping people lose weight.

Almost thirty years after we founded the program, I am the Sanford I. Weill Professor of Metabolic Research at Weill Cornell Medicine where I direct the Comprehensive Weight Control Center. We are making great strides in understanding what a complex disorder obesity is. What has become evident is that being unable to lose excess weight is not a question of willpower or motivation—it is a medical problem that involves your genes, your brain, your fat cells, and your hormones. We now know that weight problems should be treated like a chronic disease in order to succeed at lifelong weight loss.

A lot has changed since we launched the program. Obesity has become a pandemic. Now, more than two-thirds of the adults in this country are overweight, and half that number—one in three people—are obese. Global estimates of obesity rates indicate that the number of adults and children with severe weight problems has doubled in the past three decades. Being overweight is so much more than a cosmetic problem. Dr. Lee Kaplan has catalogued more than sixty illnesses that are the direct result of accumulating too much fat—breast cancer, liver disease, arthritis, pancreatitis, asthma, depression, infertility, sexual dysfunction, to name only a few of the conditions that can be caused or exacerbated by being overweight. And that's on top of the diseases that are commonly connected to obesity, such as diabetes, heart disease, high blood pressure, and stroke. The estimated annual health care costs of obesity-related illness are $190.2 billion, nearly 21 percent of yearly medical spending in the United States. Childhood obesity is responsible for $14 billion in direct medical costs. Obesity-related medical costs are expected to rise significantly as today's overweight children become overweight adults. A Cornell study reported that an obese person spends on average $2,741 more on medical care annually than a person of normal weight. If it were any other problem, we would be declaring a national health emergency. Effective weight management has clearly become our number-one health priority.

The front line of defense against the obesity epidemic rests with primary care doctors, yet fewer than 5 percent of physicians are treating obesity and excess weight in their patients. Instead, these overworked doctors tend to focus on treatable conditions such as high blood pressure and type 2 diabetes. Even though they realize that weight is the cause of much of the patients' problems, primary care physicians often relegate weight problems to the bottom of the list, because there are no wonder drugs or a standard protocol that works for every patient.

My professional focus has been on state of the art research and developing treatments to help people better manage their weight. I have performed, designed, or supervised more than sixty weight loss studies and consult regularly with other innovative researchers around the world. I have treated thousands of people trying to lose weight, working with them to find the most effective dietary, behavioral, lifestyle, and medical approaches for lasting weight loss. Doctors from all over the world refer their "toughest" patients to me—those patients who are usually between 50 and 150 pounds overweight. I help many of them drop an average of 15 to 20 percent of their initial weight, the amount they would expect to lose if they opted for lap band surgery. In addition to my practice and research,

I am getting the message out to health care providers and educating them on how to deal with this growing health care crisis.

I want to make our weight management strategies available to you. Whether you are ten pounds overweight or fifty, weighing too much can hurt you and could eventually make you sick. If you have tried diet after diet to lose weight, my message is to not give up. In my practice, I measure success one pound at a time. I have seen the program work for our patients, and believe it can work for you. With simple changes in the way you eat and move, your weight can drop, putting you on the road to good health.

*Louis J. Aronne, M.D.*

# Have You Ever Noticed that Your Weight Goes Up, But Won't Go Down?

AFTER THE AGE OF THIRTY, most Americans put on ten pounds a decade—a pound a year. A pound a year may not seem like much, but the gain is insidious and can add up before you even realize it. You do not have to remain stuck in a weight gain pattern that keeps spiraling upward. You can lose weight and maintain the loss. If you are like our patients, you have tried many diets and met with some success, only to gain back the weight you lost and more. Chances are there is nothing you would rather do than lose weight, but nothing seems to work long term. It's easy to become discouraged and to blame a lack of self-control for your inability to lose weight. After all, you were able to drop more weight than you expected during the two weeks you spent on the latest crash diet, but you couldn't keep it up and fell back into old habits. *The Change Your Biology Diet* can make yo-yo dieting a thing of the past.

I can say with authority that being overweight is not simply a matter of willpower failures or bad habits, but a medical problem with medical solutions. The availability of inexpensive, tasty, high-calorie, high-fat, high-carb food does play a role, as does not getting enough of the right exercise, but the dynamics of weight gain are far more complex than calories in/calories out. After decades of denying a physiological basis for obesity, research has shown that a number of interconnected systems contribute to slowing metabolism and increasing fat storage. Part 1 of *The Change Your Biology Diet* will give you an understanding of what is happening in your body that promotes weight gain and makes it hard to lose those extra pounds. I am going to give you a comprehensive picture of the internal biological processes that drive your weight up and put the brakes on weight loss. When our patients know the science behind their weight gain and why they are having difficulty losing those additional pounds, I believe they find it easier to comply with our weight loss program. As a result, they are more successful. They backslide less often, and, when they do, they can get right back on track, because they understand where the problems are.

Shame and guilt are not part of the program. The underlying message of recent findings is that your weight gain is not your fault. Genetics are part of the picture, but the newly emerging field of epigenetics is showing that what you have inherited is not your destiny. Though it is early, it appears that what you eat affects which of your genes turn on and which turn off. I examine the factors in modern life that contribute to the obesity epidemic. From medications with weight gain side effects to not getting enough sleep, from endocrine disruptors in the environment to the rise in the use of air-conditioning, I discuss the many causes of weight gain that often go undetected. So many factors are at play to produce the alarming prevalence of weight problems.

We have made substantial breakthroughs in understanding the biology of weight gain and weight loss resistance. Recent studies show conclusively that having difficulty controlling your weight reflects disrupted communication in your body. The food that you eat has a direct physical effect on your brain. Your body isn't designed to handle too much highly processed, starchy food. Poor eating habits actually damage your brain and appetite feedback system. Food addiction also plays a role in the obesity epidemic. Processed foods—filled with sugar, salt, and fat—are engineered to be addictive. Eating too much processed food stimulates the brain's reward pathways, making you need more food to feel satisfied. Understanding the mechanics of these alterations in your brain should make it easier to change the way you eat. Knowing what is going on biochemically in your body should give you all the motivation you need to follow the smart weight loss program you will find in these pages.

We have made a major shift in our thinking about the function of fat cells. We used to think fat cells were passive storage vessels. Now we know that fat cells are endocrine organs that produce dozens of hormones. I will explain the complex interactions of some of these hormones and the biochemical factors that prevent you from losing weight. With this information on how your body controls weight, you will know what you are up against. You will be ready to take action to combat the forces that have kept you from achieving your goal. The motto in my office is: never give up. What's the alternative? Gaining more weight?

Part 2 presents the program that we use here at the Comprehensive Weight Control Center at the Weill Cornell Medical College. I have to warn you that the Change Your Biology Diet is the antithesis of the fast, dramatic weight loss chronicled on reality TV shows. Severely overweight people on those shows can lose twenty pounds in a week by using extreme measures like not drinking water for days before weigh-ins or exercising five hours every day. These shows set up unrealistic expectations that can result in frustration and resignation.

I am opposed to fad diets, which are ultimately destructive, because people give up after repeatedly failing to keep off the weight they lost. People who have been yo-yo dieting for years come to see me in despair, saying, "I've tried everything." But they have been trying "magic bullet" diets that make big promises and have no scientific basis. If they eat an 800-calorie asparagus diet, they will lose weight. The fact is that no one can battle the extreme hunger of such a restrictive diet for long. Rather than sweating in a sauna for hours and exercising to exhaustion, my patients learn to practice other habits that help them dial down their appetites. Most of the people I treat do not lose ten pounds in ten days, but they do lose weight steadily and keep it off. My mission is to help my patients adopt long-term improvements in habits, tastes, and lifestyle that help them to control their weight.

I am very practical about losing weight and do not believe that driving yourself too hard is effective. If a diet is too restrictive, there is no way anyone can keep it up for long, which is why so many popular diets do not produce lasting weight loss. As people gradually revert to their old way of eating, their weight goes back up, sometimes higher than where they started. I suggest a way to eat that we believe will actually allow your brain to repair itself and your hormones to work as they should. A low-glycemic, low-carb, high-protein diet will keep your energy steady and turn on your fullness switch. To get you ready for the program, I explain the Breakthrough Dozen: 12 Proven Strategies for Successful Weight Control. Our research shows that when people adopt these habits they can reduce their biological tendency to gain weight.

The fact is that the best weight loss program is the one *you* like the most. If the diet is easy to follow, you are more likely to stick with it. If the diet is customized to solve your specific issues, you're more likely to comply. I am offering you two diets in this book. If one doesn't work for you, the other should. We'll teach you how to make them both flexible and exciting over the long run.

The Quick Start Change Your Biology Diet is a six-week, three-stage program that uses protein shakes for a meal or two a day to jump-start weight loss. If you do not like protein shakes or feel deprived with meal replacements, then the Two-Stage Change Your Biology Diet is for you. This low-carb, low-glycemic eating plan should get your appetite center running well again, and you should be satisfied eating less food. Stage 1 is Weight Control; stage 2 is a Lock In Weight Loss Plan that allows two servings of bread or starch a day. It is just not realistic to expect you to live without bread, potatoes, and pasta forever. I know I could not do it. I will explain the importance of portion control and food timing when you reintroduce some simple carbs to your diet. Stage 2 gives you a way to eat for the rest of your life. To make your transition to healthy eating easy, you will also find 14 Days of Change Your Biology meal plans and recipes.

Changing the way you eat is much more effective for weight loss than exercise, but I am not giving you a pass. You still need to move more, starting with getting out of that chair or off that couch. Simply standing more often during the day can help you lose weight and improve your health. As you will learn, being sedentary can take a terrible toll on your health. You might be surprised to know that adding more "everyday" movement throughout the day is more beneficial than running on a treadmill. You might spend forty minutes on a treadmill, but what are you doing the remaining twenty-three hours and twenty minutes? Moving more all day long has to become a habit.

For long-term weight maintenance, breaking through plateaus, and reversing fullness resistance, you have to move. Many of you will be relieved to hear that you are not required to exercise for hours on end on the program. In fact, there are much more efficient and effective ways to build exercise into your life. I recommend a two-step approach to exercise—lifestyle movement and high-intensity strength training—and explain why. Adam Zickerman, a high-intensity workout pioneer, author of the *New York Times* best-seller *Power of 10*, and owner of InForm Fitness with branches in New York City, Long Island, California, Virginia, and Colorado along with a mobile gym, has designed three at-home high-intensity resistance workouts specially for this book to help you build muscle. The first workout is a beginner's introduction to high-intensity resistance training, the second progresses you to a more challenging level, and the third hits a high intensity peak. You can do the eight exercises in each of these workouts in less than ten minutes, and you only have to do the workout twice a week. In twenty minutes a week, you will be building muscle mass. One of the reasons this is so important is that lean muscle burns more calories than fat. Every pound of muscle in your body burns thirty-five to fifty calories a day, even when you're not moving. As you age, you lose muscle. Resistance training will maintain your lean muscle mass and will make you a healthy, calorie-burning machine. That's worth twenty minutes of exercise a week, isn't it?

Part 3, Beyond Diet and Exercise, covers medical treatments to assist weight loss when lifestyle changes alone are not working. Just as being overweight used to be viewed as evidence of a lack of willpower, weight loss medication was considered an unhealthy crutch. Those days are over. You do not have to feel guilty or like a failure if you can't lose weight with lifestyle approaches alone. If you have diabetes and your blood sugar can't be controlled, you would take medication. The same thing goes for high blood pressure, high cholesterol, or heart disease. Obesity is no different. As you already know, being overweight can raise the risk for just about every disease on the planet. I give you guidelines for when using weight loss medications makes sense. I cover the various medications on the market, how they work, their potential benefit, possible side effects, and the type of person each is best for. This chapter will provide you with enough information to have an informed conversation with your health care providers.

Though most people can lose weight and dramatically improve their health without surgery, some people, for whom lifestyle approaches in combination with prescription medications don't do the job, opt for surgery. Lap band, sleeve gastrectomy, and gastric bypass surgery are the most frequently used procedures. I explain the surgeries, describe the pros and cons of each, the expected outcomes, and the best candidates for each method. I discuss new procedures we have begun to perform, including the vBloc vagal nerve stimulator, endoscopic sleeve gastroplasty, and Orbera and ReShape intragastric balloons, which I believe represent significant advances.

One of the benefits of my position is that we are at the forefront of the weight management field. Our own research is helping to develop treatments of the future, but we also get to review the work of my brilliant colleagues everywhere. Throughout this book, I report on the latest breakthroughs and areas of future research. We are up against an epidemic that is destroying the health of millions of people globally. Research to understand what is behind the catastrophic rise in obesity and what we can do to promote weight loss is a top priority.

If you are overweight or obese, the time to do something about it is now. Prevention is a better path than trying to restore the good health you have lost. If you are already experiencing health complications from being overweight, I have some good news for you. You don't have to lose that much weight to improve your health.

# PART 1

# It's Not Your Fault

# CHAPTER 1

# A Plan that Works

NO ONE WANTS TO BE OVERWEIGHT. In our celebrity-obsessed society, we are bombarded with images of impossibly thin or voluptuous women and sculpted men with washboard abs. These idealized images of beauty are not good for anyone's self-esteem and can be devastating for people who are overweight. Internalizing today's standard of beauty, people who weigh more can feel unappealing, ashamed, and frustrated regardless of how many pounds overweight they are.

To add to their own image problems, society stigmatizes people who are heavier. They are judged to be lazy, incompetent, and lacking in self-discipline and intelligence, because they cannot control their weight. My patients tell me that they face prejudice and discrimination every day — on the job, in social situations, in education, and even from health care professionals. If they are severely obese, they may be subjected to looks, stares, and comments about their size. Overweight children are teased and bullied and are the last ones to be picked for the team. People struggle to lose weight, because no one wants to feel inferior or be the object of contempt. They are willing to try anything to slim down.

I see the frustration my new patients have experienced when they first come to my office. By the time we meet, many of them have tried everything they could think of, every fad diet that came along, without dropping those excess pounds and keeping them off. I am glad that I can help them break that disheartening cycle with a flexible plan that helps them to achieve their goals.

## Mondo Diet

In 2012, an estimated 108 million American adults, roughly half of the adult population, were dieting. A typical dieter tries to lose weight four times a year. A huge industry has sprung up to serve this needy market. Last year, the diet industry earned $46 billion on products including gym memberships, weight loss programs, and diet sodas, to name just a few items. *Forbes* reports that two-thirds of American dieters regained all their lost weight within a year and 97 percent had put it all back on in five years. That backsliding phenomenon means that the diet market is self-renewing and continues to grow. The diet industry is more than ready to flood the market with new fads, products, programs, and regimens to satisfy the increasing demand. Our culture has become "mondo diet."

Today, the buzzwords seem to be "juice fasts" and "gluten-free." Both are supported by burgeoning businesses. All sorts of people are selling prepackaged "cleanses," and most supermarkets have special aisles selling a wide choice of gluten-free products. You might lose weight if you only consume fresh-pressed juice and some raw vegetables for a few days, but take a look at what goes into those juices. When fruit is turned into juice, the sugars found in the fruit become readily absorbable. Very few juices are made only from green vegetables. Sweet fruit and vegetables are used to make the juice palatable, and the resulting sugar content can be high. Besides, you can't stay on a juice fast for long. How much do you think a few days of fasting will actually help with your weight problem?

Eating gluten-free is all the rage now, but the long-term effect of doing so is not likely to help you reduce your weight. Gluten is a protein found in grains like wheat, rye, and barley. One percent

Lisa, who had just graduated from college, and her mother, Jill, came for a consultation. Lisa had been gaining weight steadily since she was fourteen, and her college years in the Midwest had been a disaster for her weight control. She was sixty pounds overweight. Jill had put Lisa on every new diet over the years. She clearly was frustrated that Lisa kept gaining weight despite her own efforts to help her. During the consultation, I learned that Lisa, whose self-esteem had suffered because of her weight problems, had been prescribed Zoloft for depression. When I told them that the medication could have contributed to her weight gain, Jill, had an aha moment. She confirmed that her daughter had put on the most weight when she was taking the highest dose of Zoloft.

As I explained to Lisa the biological processes behind her weight problem and the reasons she had so much trouble losing, a look of relief washed over her face, and she started to cry. Jill's face fell. Though no words were spoken, it was clear that there had been considerable conflict between daughter and mother. Jill, who had only been doing her best, put her arm around her daughter and apologized for being so hard on her day in and day out. Understanding the physical root of Lisa's struggle put her problem in perspective for both of them. I was offering Lisa a different approach to weight control, and we would fight weight loss resistance together.

I cannot tell you how often scenes like this are played out in my office at the Weight Control Center. Patients who have been struggling for years only to be defeated by their biology are finally able to release feelings of guilt and self-contempt and direct their energy to handling a disease. We restore patients' hope and don't give up until we have results.

of Americans have celiac disease, a serious immune condition that causes the small intestine to become inflamed when gluten is eaten, resulting in gastrointestinal discomfort and eventual damage to intestinal walls. Six to seven percent of Americans are believed to have nonceliac gluten intolerance or sensitivity, though a test for it does not exist. Gluten intolerance is not an autoimmune disorder nor an allergic reaction. Consuming gluten for those sensitive to it leads to digestive issues, fatigue, and brain fog. New research suggests that gluten alone may not be responsible for such symptoms. It appears that a group of slowly digested carbohydrates known as FODMAPS (fermentable oligosaccharides, disaccharides, monosaccharides, and polyols), lactose, and certain preservatives in processed food could produce the same symptoms. Nevertheless, people believe they will benefit if they eliminate gluten from their diets. Sales of gluten-free products are estimated to hit $15 billion by 2016—a 50 percent jump over 2013 numbers.

When people start to eat gluten-free, they tend to stop eating re-fined carbohydrates, which could lead to weight loss. But then they discover the "gluten-free store" and reintroduce cookies, crackers, pasta, pancakes, and pizza to their diets in gluten-free form. The truth is that gluten-free products can be as high in calories as conven-tional processed food and sometimes higher. Check the carbohydrate and sugar content on the food labels of these products. Gluten-free does not necessarily mean you are eating healthy, diet-friendly food. When it comes to losing weight, eating a box of gluten-free cookies is just as bad for you as eating a box of cookies made with flour. Don't get swept up by the notion that the abundance of gluten-free prod-ucts available means they will make a big difference in your weight and how you feel.

People, looking for quick fixes and easy answers, are eager to try diets with big promises. The diet marketing machine, fueled by word of mouth, drives chronic dieters to lose their common sense. Even af-ter repeated disappointments, they are ready to try the latest fad diet and buy low-carb, sugar-free, gluten-free, no-fat, vegan products for weight loss and improved health without studying the food label and ingredients.

Admittedly, it is easier to follow a diet that lays everything out for you than to be responsible for your own healthy eating plan, but usually fad diets cannot and should not be sustained. I admire the optimism involved in believing you'll succeed the next time, be-cause you'll try harder—despite having failed time and time again. You want to believe that there is an answer out there, one way to lose weight. You have convinced yourself that by following a very restricted, deprivation diet for two weeks, twenty-one days, or a month, your weight problems will be over. If you met with initial success in the past, you might remember when you felt in control. You lost weight, and you felt great. You are ready to replicate that feeling and believe that it will last this time. You remain hopeful every time you try a new diet.

# A Brief History of Diets

I've compiled a list of popular diets of the past hundred years to give you an idea of the extremes to which people have gone in the attempt to lose weight. Some of the diets might seem comical now, but many were taken seriously at the time. You'll see that some of the diets have been recycled decades later, proving that weight loss plans go in and out of style.

The truth is that if you reduce your caloric intake sufficiently, you will lose weight, but you don't want to jeopardize your health while doing so. Though I am sure people went on diets as far back as Greek and Roman times, those regimens were primarily designed to promote health rather than manage weight. The diets that follow reflect the trends in weight management plans and some of the real misses in the two-hundred-year war against weight gain.

**1820: The cider vinegar and water diet** has been attributed to Lord Byron, who ate a restricted diet to maintain his Romantic poet look. His daily intake is reported to have been a thin slice of bread, a few potatoes soaked in vinegar, a cup of tea, and water.

**1825: Jean-Anthelme Brillat-Savarin** was the father of the **low-carbohydrate diet.** An epicure, he wrote *The Physiology of Taste.* He believed that sugar and flour were the root cause of obesity.

**1830: Graham's diet** was a vegetarian, whole-grain regimen created by Sylvester Graham, the inventor of the graham cracker.

**1863: Banting's low-carbohydrate diet**—William Banting, an obese undertaker, lost weight by limiting refined carbohydrates in his diet. The name Banting became synonymous with dieting at the time.

**1897: Raw foods**—Swiss physician Maximilian Bircher-Benner claimed he cured himself of jaundice by eating raw apples. He did a number of experiments and ended up opening a treatment center in Zurich where he advanced his theory that consuming raw fruits and vegetables was the healthiest way to eat.

**1900: The tapeworm diet**—Beef tapeworm cysts were swallowed in the form of a pill, and the tapeworm developed in the intestines. When the dieter was down to the desired weight, antiparasitic pills would take care of the tapeworm. The possible side effects—seizures, meningitis, and dementia—must have dissuaded many from this radical and revolting weight loss method.

**1903: Fletcherizing**—Horace Fletcher, known as "The Great Masticator," stressed the importance of chewing your food until it was liquefied—about thirty-two times—before swallowing. He recommended spitting out the solids that remained.

**1917: Lulu Hunt Peters' calorie counter**—An M.D., Dr. Peters struggled with her own weight and began to count calories. She promoted calorie counting for weight loss through her newspaper column and diet books. The calorie had been "invented" by chemists about fifty years earlier as a way to measure the amount of chemical energy in a substance.

**1925: The cigarette diet**—This diet was so popular Lucky Strike cigarettes advertised, "Reach for a Lucky instead of a sweet."

**1928: Inuit meat and fat diet**—This is one of the original hunter-gatherer diets. Since the Inuits are unable to grow crops on the frozen tundra, they subsist on wild fish, blubber, and game. Vilhjalmur Stefansson, an Artic explorer, ate Inuit-style for five years during two expeditions. On his return, he spent a year on an Americanized version of the diet under medical supervision at Bellevue Hospital to convince skeptics that it was healthy.

**1930s: Slimming soaps**—The promise of washing away fat while bathing appealed to many women. "Fatoff," "Fat-O-No," and "La-Mar Reducing Soap" made claims that lathering up with these products would have a slimming effect. Slimming soaps are still being sold today.

**1930: Dr. Stoll's Diet Aid**—Dr. Stoll sold one of the first liquid diets through beauty parlors.

**1930: Hay diet**—Dr. William Howard Hay came up with one of the first food combination diets, which prohibited consuming starches and proteins at the same meal.

**1934: Bananas and skim milk diet**—Created by Dr. George Harrop, this diet was publicized by the United Fruit Company.

**1950: The grapefruit diet or Hollywood diet** claims that grapefruit contains a fat-burning enzyme. While eating reduced calories, the dieter has a half grapefruit before every meal. This diet is still used today.

**1950: The cabbage and fruit diet** (except bananas) is a short-term diet described by its name. This diet is low-calorie, low-fat, low-protein, and low on essential nutrients. The quick weight loss is mostly fluids. This diet has made a comeback.

**1954: Dr. A. T. W. Simeons,** a British endocrinologist practicing in Rome, published *Pounds and Inches*. His diet uses the hormone **hCG (human chorionic gonadotropin)**, which is found in the urine of pregnant women. A daily injection of hCG in addition to consuming 500 calories a day from a list of allowed foods is said to result in losing thirty pounds in a month. hCG has only been approved as a way to treat infertility, not as a way to lose body fat. Ten studies have shown no additional benefit of hCG over and above the diet alone and a daily shot of a placebo. Of course you will lose weight if you eat only 500 calories a day for a month. How can hCG be sold and marketed for this purpose when it is no better than a placebo and the FDA has made it clear that it is not approved for weight loss and does not work? Beats me.

**1960: The Zen Macrobiotic Diet**—George Ohsawa, a Japanese philosopher who wanted to integrate Zen Buddhism with Asian medicine and Western philosophy and medicine, developed this diet. Ohsawa believed simplicity in diet was the key to good health. This vegetarian diet consists of whole grains, cereals, and vegetables. Gwyneth Paltrow resurrected this diet most recently.

**1961: The Calories Don't Count Diet**—An obstetrician named Herman Taller developed this diet after losing weight himself. He advocated the total avoidance of carbohydrates in the form of sugars, refined, and processed foods and the unlimited consumption of fat and meat protein. The FDA charged him for unsubstantiated claims.

**1963: Weight Watchers**—Jean Nidetch created a point system that allowed dieters to eat anything they wanted as long as they kept track of the point value of the food they had eaten and did not exceed their point limit for the day. The diet remains popular worldwide to this day.

**1964: The Drinking Man's Diet**—Robert Cameron wrote a little pamphlet on this low-carb diet that sold 2.4 million copies and was translated into thirteen languages. The diet involves consuming alcohol and richly sauced meats and fish. It's low carb with a twist. Think *Mad Men*.

**1976: The Sleeping Beauty Diet**—Elvis is rumored to have tried this diet. Dieters would be heavily sedated and sleep for several days eating little and in some cases receiving IV fluids. The operating theory was that you can't eat if you're asleep. Some spas in Europe use a variation of this diet—a real "rest cure."

Since the '70s, we have had the Pritikin Program, the Caveman and Paleo diets, the Scarsdale Diet, Dean Ornish's Low-Fat Diet, The Zone, Raw Food Diet, Eating Right for Your Type, the fasts and the juice cleanses. There seem to be at least one breakout diet a year.

I have listed all these diets—from the sublime to the ridiculous—to make a point: people are always looking for a new solution to their weight problems and will latch on to the latest diet with renewed hope. You would think in all this time it would have become clear that fad diets don't work for the long haul. If any of these diets really worked, there would be no need to keep coming up with novelty diets or putting a new spin on old weight loss programs. In the meantime, obesity rates keep climbing.

Several telltale signs can help you identify fad diets that are not long-term solutions to weight problems. Diets designed to sell a product are obviously suspect. Fad diets promise a quick fix, one that is too good to be true. A weight management program should have realistic goals. If you've ever tried a magic bullet diet and did not maintain the weight you lost, you should be able to recognize another one. Being "on a diet" and then gradually returning to your former eating habits will not work. If you want to lose weight and keep it off, you have to commit to making permanent changes in the way you eat.

You also have to consider the sources and references to see if the diet plan is solidly grounded in science. Fad diets are often based on testimonials, a single poorly done study, or oversimplified conclusions drawn from a more complex study. Look at the sources and references to gauge whether the plan is based on peer-reviewed studies and solid science.

It is not a good sign if a diet eliminates one or more food groups. Neither is it promising if a weight loss plan focuses on a single food—cabbage soup, leeks, bananas, for example. There is a built-in limit to how long you will be able to eat that way. When you "finish" the diet, it usually doesn't take long to backslide. These diets are not providing you with a way to eat when you are not starving yourself. You cannot "cure" this chronic disease without changing how you eat all the time and making regular exercise a part of your life.

# The Complications of Being Overweight

Aside from aesthetics, health problems associated with being overweight or the desire to prevent illnesses from developing are important motivations for wanting to slim down. Not only does being overweight affect the quality of your life every day, but those excess pounds can cut years off your life. **More than sixty illnesses have been associated with increased body fat.** It's that simple. Here are some of the complications associated with obesity:

> **Cardiovascular disease** is the number-one cause of death for men and women in the United States. As your weight rises, so does your risk for cardiovascular disease. Being overweight or obese can promote the buildup of plaque in your arteries, which can lead to high blood pressure and an increased risk of heart attack, stroke, or kidney failure. Plaque in the coronary arteries can narrow the blood flow to the heart, resulting in chest pain, known as angina, heart attack, heart failure, and stroke.

Natalie had been a chubby teenager, overweight since puberty. She gained forty pounds her first year of college. Her periods had become irregular, and she developed acne. She repeatedly tried to lose weight. She'd take off five to ten pounds but would always put the weight back on.

Now thirty-four years old, she weighed 172 pounds with a BMI of 29.5. She had been trying to get pregnant for a year. Her weight was affecting her hormone balance, and her hormones were affecting her weight. She could not detect if she was ovulating. Before going through a battery of fertility tests, her doctor recommended that she lose weight to see if it would help, and recommended the Comprehensive Weight Control Center.

I gave Natalie a prescription for metformin, and she agreed to follow the Change Your Biology Diet. She was highly motivated. She lost forty-five pounds in four months. Her weight was down to 132, and her BMI was 22.7. She arrived at a follow-up appointment elated. Natalie had just discovered she was pregnant.

**Type 2 diabetes** is the leading cause of early death, heart disease, stroke, kidney disease, and blindness. Most people who have type 2 diabetes are overweight and have developed insulin resistance, which means that muscle and liver cells do not respond to normal levels of insulin, the pancreatic hormone that carries glucose, or blood sugar, into cells. As a result, glucose levels in the bloodstream go up and stay up, stimulating the pancreas to keep pumping out insulin. Diabetes is diagnosed when glucose gets above 125 mg/dl fasting, or the test of long-term blood sugar, the HbA1c is above 6.4%. Prediabetes begins at a blood glucose of 100 mg/dl and an HbA1c of 5.6%.

**Abnormal blood lipids or fats** are related to weight. People with excessive body fat have increased triglyceride levels and LDL (bad) cholesterol and decreased HDL (good) cholesterol. This combination creates optimal conditions for developing heart disease.

**Metabolic syndrome** affects almost 34 percent of adults in this country. It has become one of the fastest-growing health problems in the United States. The syndrome consists of a cluster of factors that raises your risk for heart disease, diabetes, and stroke. These risk factors tend to occur together. Metabolic syndrome is diagnosed if you have three of the following conditions:

- Having an apple shape with a large waistline. A waist measurement of more than 40 inches for men and more than 35 inches for women is unhealthy. Having extra fat in your middle is a greater risk factor for heart disease than having extra fat elsewhere, such as your hips.

- High triglyceride level: 150 mg/dL or higher (or take medication to treat the condition)

- Low HDL cholesterol level: 40 or lower mg/dL for men and 50 or lower mg/dL for women (or take medication)

- High blood pressure: 130/85 or higher (or take medication)

- High fasting blood sugar: 100 mg/DL or higher (or take medication to treat diabetes)

**Cancer risk,** most specifically for colon, breast, endometrial, and prostate cancer, is raised if you are overweight or obese.

**Sexual dysfunction, reproductive hormonal abnormalities, and infertility** are associated with being overweight in men.

**Polycystic ovary syndrome** is the most common hormonal disorder in reproductive-age women. A majority of patients with this diagnosis are overweight. Characterized by irregular menstrual cycles and ovarian cysts, the syndrome is a leading cause of infertility and a risk factor in developing diabetes.

**Osteoarthritis** occurs in the knees, hips, and lower back when the tissue that protects the joints wears away. Extra weight causes wear and tear on the joints, which can result in pain. Even arthritis of the hands is more common due to excessive inflammation.

**Asthma and obesity** have been linked. Studies have shown that weight gain increases the risk of asthma, and weight loss improves the illness. Adults and children with obesity have more chronic low-grade systemic inflammation, and asthma is a chronic inflammatory disease. In addition, the lungs of obese people may be underexpanded, which causes them to take smaller breaths. As a result, their lung airways are narrow and prone to irritation.

**Sleep apnea** is a disorder in which you have pauses in your breath while you sleep. Excess fat stored around the neck may narrow the airway, making it hard to breathe while you are lying down. This can be a severe health problem, associated with depression, diabetes, erectile dysfunction, and heart failure, and is often misdiagnosed.

**Gallstones,** which are mostly made of cholesterol, can form in the gallbladder, causing stomach or back pain. If you are overweight, you are at increased risk of developing gallstones. Of note, rapid weight loss may also increase the risk of forming gallstones.

**Dementia** and having too much weight around your middle are connected. Excess belly fat during midlife may increase the risk of developing dementia, including Alzheimer's disease, in old age. Belly fat threatens your brain.

You would have to be living in a cave to avoid knowing about some of the health risks of being overweight. Consider the above list a wake-up call. If you want to maintain your health or reduce the problems you already have, you have to take charge of what you eat and how much you move to control your weight. *The Change Your Biology Diet* gives you a science-based plan to jump-start weight loss and optimize your health.

# It Doesn't Take that Much to Turn It Around

When you think about losing weight, you probably start with a target weight in mind, an ideal number you dream of seeing when you get on the scale. I advise you to take smaller steps. If you set your goals in small, achievable increments, you are less likely to become frustrated. **You will start to see the benefits of weight reduction with a loss of just 5 to 10 percent of your body weight.** If you weigh 180 pounds, you could see health improvements if you drop nine to eighteen pounds. Many complications of obesity improve or are prevented from developing with this small a reduction in weight.

If you lose between 5 and 10 percent of your body weight, you can:

- Increase your good HDL cholesterol by 5 points.

- Decrease triglycerides significantly, an average of 40 mg/dl.

- Losing just ten to twelve pounds can reduce the risk of developing diabetes by 60 percent.

If you lose 10 percent or more of your weight, you can:

- Lower your risk factors for cardiovascular disease. One study showed that with each 10 percent increase in weight, there was a 30 percent increase in coronary heart disease (CHD) in men, while a 10 percent weight loss resulted in a 20 percent reduction in CHD in men.

- Reduce the risk of diabetes 80 percent or more.

- Significantly reduce inflammatory substances circulating in the blood, reducing inflammation in the blood vessels and the risk of coronary artery disease.

- Improve knee function if you have osteoarthritis. Studies have shown that patients with osteoarthritis in the knee have improved function by 28 percent with a 10 percent weight loss. Being only ten pounds overweight increases the force on the knee by thirty to sixty pounds with each step. That extra weight causes a lot of wear and tear on the knee joint. For every pound of weight lost, there is a four-pound reduction in the load exerted on the knee with each step taken. Every eleven-pound weight loss reduces the risk of knee osteoarthritis by more than 50 percent. Being overweight has similar effects on your hip joints as well. Many studies have shown that weight loss can reduce the pain of knee and hip arthritis.

- Reduce hot flashes caused by menopause. The more weight you lose, the more hot flash relief you are likely to experience.

- May improve mild sleep apnea. It will take somewhat more weight loss to reduce severe sleep apnea.

- Being overweight is at the root of 25 to 30 percent of high blood pressure. Losing a small amount of weight will decrease both systolic and diastolic blood pressure by an average of 5 mmHG.

- Decreases insulin levels, helps to reverse insulin resistance, and reduces the amount of abdominal fat that results from the condition.

- Reduce lower back pain. Research has shown that the risk of lower back pain increases as BMI (body mass index) increases. Adding just twenty minutes of moderate exercise a day can lower an overweight person's risk of low back pain by 17 percent. Adding exercise to your life is part of the program.

Matt, a forty-three-year-old college history professor, is a big man. He's six feet tall, 271 pounds, BMI 36.2, and has a forty-eight-inch waist. He had put on twenty pounds in the past year. The father of four children, he was distressed by developing health problems. He had been diagnosed with fatty liver disease, high triglycerides, and low HDL (good cholesterol). His triglycerides were three times higher than normal. His parents had a history of hypertension, type 2 diabetes, and hyperlipidemia, and he did not want to follow in their footsteps. When we did tests, we found that he was prediabetic. Matt desperately wanted to reverse his metabolic syndrome.

When he described his lifestyle, we could see some immediate changes that had to be made. He would grab a quick, high-carb breakfast, skip lunch, and be out of control with his eating at night. Between the demands of a large family and his teaching schedule, his days were packed. Doing his own research and reading students' papers kept him up late at night. He averaged five hours of sleep a night, which was not enough restorative sleep for him. He could not find the time to use the state-of-the-art gym at the university, and he was too exhausted anyway. Instead, he started walking three times a week—and made it family time. He began to follow a low-glycemic diet and made sure to eat a protein-rich breakfast and filled up on salad at his other meals. Matt makes sure to eat his vegetables and protein before carbs and tells me this strategy works to fill him up.

When other options produced little weight loss, he started taking a low dose of liraglutide (Saxenda) by injection and his weight began to fall. He was down to 247, a loss of twenty-one pounds. Even more important in a short time—only six weeks—his health had improved. His blood sugar levels, liver function, and triglycerides were excellent. When he saw what a few changes could do to relieve him of his health problems, he had no trouble believing that his continued efforts would get him to a healthy weight. He resolved to take up high-intensity weight training to build lean muscle and lock in his weight loss.

As much as 90 percent of all diabetes, 80 percent of heart disease, and 60 percent of cancers are preventable with healthier lifestyles and normal body weights. Rather than relying solely on medical treatment for these diseases, we are now taking a "weight-centric" approach, a term I've coined, to managing them. Taking off excess pounds will improve your health and can reverse existing conditions.

My overview of the benefits of losing weight should go a long way to convincing you that it is worth the effort. You probably don't need to be persuaded, but knowing how quickly your body can respond to even a modest weight loss should be encouraging. You can measure the improvements in your health just as you keep track of the weight you have lost. Once you begin to correct health problems, you will feel so much better—physically and emotionally. When you take off some weight and eat right, you can experience a boost in energy and mood that can propel you to eat in a way that supports further weight loss.

# Is Your Weight a Threat to Your Health?

There are a number of ways to determine if you are overweight, and if so, how high a risk you have of developing weight-related complications such as diabetes, hypertension, and cardiovascular disease. We are refining the best way to determine if you are in a danger zone with your weight. Three measurements will give you a full picture: BMI measures total fat; waist circumference measures internal fat; and the ratio of your waist to your height, a newer measure, is an effective way to estimate the risk for cardiovascular disease, diabetes, and other metabolic issues.

## BODY MASS INDEX (BMI)

As a starting point, you should consider your body mass index (BMI), a calculation based on your height and weight that is a general measure of obesity. There are several calculators online that will save you from having to do the math, including:

www.nhlbi.nih.gov/health/educational/lose_wt/BMI/bmicalc .htm

www.cdc.gov/healthyweight/assessing/bmi/adult_bmi/english _bmi_calculator/bmi_calculator.html

| BMI (Body Mass Index) | | | | | | | | | | | | | | | | | | | | | |
|---|---|---|---|---|---|---|---|---|---|---|---|---|---|---|---|---|---|---|---|---|---|
| | 19 | 20 | 21 | 22 | 23 | 24 | 25 | 26 | 27 | 28 | 29 | 30 | 31 | 32 | 33 | 34 | 35 | 36 | 37 | 38 | 39 | 40 |
| 58 | 91 | 96 | 100 | 105 | 110 | 115 | 119 | 124 | 129 | 134 | 138 | 143 | 148 | 153 | 158 | 162 | 167 | 172 | 177 | 181 | 186 | 191 |
| 59 | 94 | 99 | 104 | 109 | 114 | 119 | 124 | 128 | 133 | 138 | 143 | 148 | 153 | 158 | 163 | 168 | 173 | 178 | 183 | 188 | 193 | 198 |
| 60 | 97 | 102 | 107 | 112 | 118 | 123 | 128 | 133 | 138 | 143 | 148 | 153 | 158 | 163 | 168 | 174 | 179 | 184 | 189 | 194 | 199 | 204 |
| 61 | 100 | 106 | 111 | 116 | 122 | 127 | 132 | 137 | 143 | 148 | 153 | 158 | 164 | 169 | 174 | 180 | 185 | 190 | 195 | 201 | 206 | 211 |
| 62 | 104 | 109 | 115 | 120 | 126 | 131 | 136 | 142 | 147 | 153 | 158 | 164 | 169 | 175 | 180 | 186 | 191 | 196 | 202 | 207 | 213 | 218 |
| 63 | 107 | 113 | 118 | 124 | 130 | 135 | 141 | 146 | 152 | 158 | 163 | 169 | 175 | 180 | 186 | 191 | 197 | 203 | 208 | 214 | 220 | 225 |
| 64 | 110 | 116 | 122 | 128 | 134 | 140 | 145 | 151 | 157 | 163 | 169 | 174 | 180 | 186 | 192 | 197 | 204 | 209 | 215 | 221 | 227 | 232 |
| 65 | 114 | 120 | 126 | 132 | 138 | 144 | 150 | 156 | 162 | 168 | 174 | 180 | 186 | 192 | 198 | 204 | 210 | 216 | 222 | 228 | 234 | 240 |
| 66 | 118 | 124 | 130 | 136 | 142 | 148 | 155 | 161 | 167 | 173 | 179 | 186 | 192 | 198 | 204 | 210 | 216 | 223 | 229 | 235 | 241 | 247 |
| 67 | 121 | 127 | 134 | 140 | 146 | 153 | 159 | 166 | 172 | 178 | 185 | 191 | 198 | 204 | 211 | 217 | 223 | 230 | 236 | 242 | 249 | 255 |
| 68 | 125 | 131 | 138 | 144 | 151 | 158 | 164 | 171 | 177 | 184 | 190 | 197 | 204 | 210 | 216 | 223 | 230 | 236 | 243 | 249 | 256 | 262 |
| 69 | 128 | 135 | 142 | 149 | 155 | 162 | 169 | 176 | 182 | 189 | 196 | 203 | 210 | 216 | 223 | 230 | 236 | 243 | 250 | 257 | 263 | 270 |
| 70 | 132 | 139 | 146 | 153 | 160 | 167 | 174 | 181 | 188 | 195 | 202 | 209 | 216 | 222 | 229 | 236 | 243 | 250 | 257 | 264 | 271 | 278 |
| 71 | 136 | 143 | 150 | 157 | 165 | 172 | 179 | 186 | 193 | 200 | 208 | 215 | 222 | 229 | 236 | 243 | 250 | 257 | 265 | 272 | 279 | 286 |
| 72 | 140 | 147 | 154 | 162 | 169 | 177 | 184 | 191 | 199 | 206 | 213 | 221 | 228 | 235 | 242 | 250 | 258 | 265 | 272 | 279 | 287 | 294 |
| 73 | 144 | 151 | 159 | 166 | 174 | 182 | 189 | 197 | 204 | 212 | 219 | 227 | 235 | 242 | 250 | 257 | 265 | 272 | 280 | 288 | 295 | 302 |
| 74 | 148 | 155 | 163 | 171 | 179 | 186 | 194 | 202 | 210 | 218 | 225 | 233 | 241 | 249 | 256 | 264 | 272 | 280 | 287 | 295 | 303 | 311 |
| 75 | 152 | 160 | 168 | 176 | 184 | 192 | 200 | 208 | 216 | 224 | 232 | 240 | 248 | 256 | 264 | 272 | 279 | 287 | 295 | 303 | 311 | 319 |
| 76 | 156 | 164 | 172 | 180 | 189 | 197 | 205 | 213 | 221 | 230 | 238 | 246 | 254 | 263 | 271 | 279 | 287 | 295 | 304 | 312 | 320 | 328 |

Height (inches) · Weight (lbs.)

The weight ranges for BMI are as follows:

**Underweight:** BMI below 18.5

**Normal:** BMI between 18.5 and 24.9

**Overweight:** BMI between 25 and 29.9

**Obese Class I (low-risk):** BMI between 30 and 34.9

**Obese Class II (moderate-risk):** BMI between 35.0 and 39.9

**Obese Class III (high-risk):** BMI over 40

Although very helpful, BMI is a limited tool and can be misleading for a number of reasons. I have had patients whose BMI indicates that they are overweight, but their cholesterol, triglycerides, blood pressure, and blood sugar are in the normal range. Their excess weight does not seem to be affecting their health, or at least not yet. Others have a BMI under 25, but have all the symptoms of metabolic syndrome. One reason for this is that the BMI reveals nothing about body composition and fat location. Someone may have a high BMI, but not have a lot of body fat. Bodybuilders and athletes can be muscular and lean but weigh a lot for their height. The extra muscle tissue can raise their BMI, causing them to be incorrectly categorized as overweight or obese. At the same time, some very inactive people have a BMI in the normal range, yet they have excess fat in comparison to their lean body mass. This can happen with the elderly, the sick, and people in poor physical condition, who have low levels of muscle and bone, which would make them weigh less. Their lower BMI may underestimate their body fat. Their risk of developing disease can be similar to that of someone with a high BMI. Considering waist circumference helps to correct these problems in interpretation.

Age is another factor that might require a shift in standard BMI levels. Older people tend to do better if they carry a little more fat on their bodies. I mean a little overweight, not a BMI over thirty. The best BMI for most elderly people is on the low end of overweight, say a BMI of twenty-five or twenty-six. Studies have shown that with age, people with a few extra pounds have a better survival rate than leaner people. We do not know why, but there is some speculation that they have more muscle mass, or that extra fat could provide reserves from which to draw on to fight off illness.

When it comes to interpreting BMI, there are ethnic differences. The Centers for Disease Control has released these obesity figures:

African Americans 47.8%

Hispanics 42.5%

White Europeans 32.6%

Asians 10.8%

Research has found that at the same BMI, Asians had more than double the risk of developing type 2 diabetes, higher risks of hypertension and cardiovascular disease, and a higher risk of dying early than white Europeans with the same BMI. Hispanics have an 85 percent greater risk, and blacks a 35 percent greater risk, of developing diabetes at the same BMI. The amount, location, and composition of body fat is a possible explanation, because, for example, Asians have 3 to 5 percent higher total body fat than white Europeans with the same BMI, while more Hispanics and blacks have a higher BMI and more body fat. The overall risk for diabetes is double in blacks and 75 percent greater in Hispanics because of the higher average BMI of those ethnic groups and 40 percent greater in Asians because of the location and size of fat cells despite a lower average BMI compared to whites.

The chart that follows is the result of one study done in New York:

| Week of: | Ethnicity | Mean BMI | Body Fat % |
| --- | --- | --- | --- |
| Male | White | 25.2 | 19.6% |
| | Black | 26.3 | 22% |
| | Asian | 23.3 | 21.3% |
| | Puerto Rican | 27.4 | 24.8% |
| Female | White | 23.3 | 30.8% |
| | Black | 28.5 | 38.2% |
| | Asian | 22.0 | 31.9% |
| | Puerto Rican | 29.4 | 40.2% |

## WAIST CIRCUMFERENCE

Adding your waist measurement is a better way to assess your health risks than with your BMI alone. To do so, women should measure at the narrowest point, men at their navel. A trim waistline is a good indication that you don't have a large buildup of visceral fat.

> The Centers for Disease Control and Prevention state that women with a waist circumference greater than thirty-five inches and men whose waists are more than forty inches may be at a greater risk of developing weight-related health problems. This risk is compounded by also having a BMI over thirty.

Where your fat is located affects your health. As waistlines grow, so do health risks. If most of your fat is around your middle rather than your hips, if you are an "apple" rather than a "pear," you are at a higher risk for heart disease, type 2 diabetes, elevated triglycerides and LDL cholesterol, and high blood pressure. The risk goes up with waist size. Your genetic makeup is partially responsible for accumulating fat around your middle. Specific genes determine how many fat cells you have and where they will settle. Lifestyle, specifically your diet and how much you exercise, contributes to the condition.

## NOT ALL BELLY FAT IS THE SAME

There are two types of abdominal fat: subcutaneous and visceral. Subcutaneous fat is the layer of fat that lies just beneath the skin and over the muscles in your entire body. This is the "pinchable" fat you can measure with calipers. Visceral fat lies beneath the muscles, deeper in the abdominal cavity. This type of fat pads the space between abdominal organs and wraps around organs such as the liver, pancreas, and intestines. Blood from visceral fat flows through the liver, bathing it in products of fat breakdown. Even slim people can have dangerous, hidden, visceral fat.

Men collect more abdominal fat than women, as seen with the prevalence of "beer bellies" that are hard to the touch. Developing central obesity starts earlier in men, sometime in adolescence. This tendency to gain weight around the middle is one of the reasons men historically have had more heart disease than women, though that is changing as obesity becomes more widespread in both sexes. In the past, women appeared not to accumulate visceral fat before menopause. For women, fat tends to collect in the hips and thighs, which offers them protection from heart disease. When a woman's estrogen level drops after menopause, her midsection can grow, contributing to health problems. A woman with a large waist is five times more likely to die of heart disease than a woman with a measurement under thirty-five inches and is two times more likely to develop gallstones. For both men and women, the proportion of fat to weight increases with middle age, as seen in "middle-age spread."

You might be wondering why abdominal fat is so bad for you. All fat cells are biologically active and operate as endocrine organs or glands, but abdominal fat cells are especially active. Belly fat churns out hormones and inflammatory substances, which profoundly affect health. Excess visceral fat disrupts hormonal balance and the way hormones function. For example, visceral fat secretes the precursor to angiotensin II, the hormone that controls blood vessel constriction and directly affects blood pressure. Too much angiotensin II can lead directly to hypertension. Visceral fat also releases inflammatory molecules on a consistent basis. It pumps out immune system chemicals, called cytokines, including tumor necrosis factor alpha and interleukin-6, which cause an inflammatory reaction that increases the risk of cardiovascular disease.

Visceral fat breaks down easily into fatty acids that flow directly into the liver. Since abdominal fat is located in the circulation of the portal vein, a blood vessel that carries blood from the gastrointestinal tract and spleen to the liver, the free fatty acids released by visceral fat travel to the liver, where they can influence the production of blood lipids or fats. Having fat around your middle is linked with higher total cholesterol, higher LDL, lower HDL, higher triglycerides, and insulin resistance.

**The good news is that it is easier to lose potentially damaging visceral fat than subcutaneous fat at your waist, which can be difficult to reduce.** Belly fat responds well to exercise and diet. No over-the-counter pills or supplements will help you lose that fat faster. There are no quick fixes, and that includes all the available exercise gear such as rollers, ab belts, and ab rockers. Spot exercise can tighten your muscles but will not get at visceral fat. Combatting abdominal fat is a matter of eating well and exercising in a way that stimulates necessary hormonal and metabolic response. One study compared groups who lost weight with diet only and those who had a program that combined diet and exercise. The group that did not exercise lost less abdominal fat than those who did moderate exercise along with changing their eating habits. Chapter 10 will show you how to make moderate exercise a part of your life and give you three high-intensity resistance training programs to help you build muscle mass in two ten-minute workouts a week.

### RATIO OF WAIST TO HEIGHT

While BMI correlates with total fat for most people and waist size correlates with internal fat, some studies are showing waist-to-height ratio to be an effective way of detecting metabolic risk in men and women. The drawback with waist circumference alone is that it does not take height into account. A thirty-four-inch waist on a woman five feet tall is different from a thirty-four-inch waist on a woman who is five feet eight.

> The weight to height ratio is easy to calculate: your waist circumference should be less than half your height.

Using this measure, the five-foot woman's waistline should be less than thirty inches, and the taller woman's should be less than thirty-four inches. Though this measure has not yet been widely accepted, making this calculation in conjunction with BMI and waist circumference will give you a personalized assessment of your weight problem, whether your health is in jeopardy, and to what degree.

• • •

From popular diets through the years to the health risks of being overweight, from the benefits of losing just 5 to 10 percent of your body weight to how visceral fat can undermine your health, this chapter is a wake-up call. It is time to make up your mind to lose those extra pounds with a sensible plan that has been proven to work. Forget about crash diets with quick results. You have to be ready to make changes in your life that will put you on the path of gradual weight loss. We have spent more than thirty years studying the most effective ways to lose weight and have designed a practical diet and exercise plan that is intentionally not hard to follow. We want you to succeed, not give up in frustration. Losing weight is challenging enough without our setting the hurdles so high that you are defeated before you begin.

The next chapter delivers an important message: it's not your fault if you are having difficulty losing weight. There are a multitude of factors in modern life that fuel the obesity epidemic. You are up against your biology as well as an environment that boosts weight gain. Let's examine some of the external causes of the prevalence of weight problems today.

CHAPTER 2

# Fattening Factors

ULTIMATELY, WEIGHT GAIN IS THE RESULT of an imbalance between calories in and calories out, or consuming more calories than you burn. Until recently, the narrow focus has been on lifestyle choices—eating too much and exercising too little. If the calories in what you eat are not converted to physical energy, they are stored as fat to provide energy reserves. Though this dynamic is undeniable, it is too simplistic an explanation for what is now an epidemic. Viewing the global rise in weight as a matter of calories in/calories out makes individuals responsible for the obesity epidemic. Those are two important explanations for why people gain weight, but there is so much more to it than that.

We are looking at the bigger picture. There are a surprising number of fattening factors in modern life that interact to fuel the ever-increasing weight gain we have witnessed during the last forty years. Remember that the weight of the most obese people is much higher than the top end of obesity in the past. To get to the root causes of the obesity epidemic and your personal struggle to manage your weight, we need to consider the genetic, physiological, environmental, social, economic, and political issues that come into play, the fattening factors that interact to drive your weight up.

Economics have a broad effect on a population's tendency to gain weight. A degree of prosperity is an enabler for obesity, and the level of prosperity doesn't have to be high for weight gain to happen. In general, greater prosperity leads to greater consumption of all products, and that includes food. Not only have we become more prosperous in the past fifty years, the population has shifted from younger to older, rural to urban. Those demographic shifts increase average weight and skew the statistics, because weight tends to go up with age and rural life is associated with more physical activity than urban life.

In addition to these broad, societal changes, there are many fattening factors that affect you as an individual.

# The Price of Convenience

In the last few decades of the twentieth century, we hit a tipping point in energy balance. The food environment shifted in ways that promoted overeating. The supply of inexpensive, high-calorie foods became almost limitless. Americans eat out or order in more than they did a few decades ago and have less control over how their food is prepared. In the '70s, government policies were put in place to increase the food supply. Farm subsidies led to an abundance of certain foods, especially corn, which resulted in lowering prices and pushing up the amount of food people ate. High-fructose corn syrup, a by-product of the food subsidies, came into use as an inexpensive sweetener.

Food manufacturing companies responded to the demands of the fast pace of modern life and developed inexpensive, convenient, easy-to-prepare food. Eighty percent of what you find in the grocery store is processed food. Supermarket shelves are packed with highly processed, prepackaged food with very long shelf lives. Highly refined foods lose nutrients in the process, so vitamins and minerals are often added along with preservatives, dyes, emulsifiers, and countless other chemicals. Since the original whole food lost flavor in processing, lots of sugar, fat, and salt have been added to make it more palatable—which is a cocktail for weight gain.

Kate worked as a coder in new development for a major search engine and loved the culture of the company. She enjoyed working with her colleagues so much that the long hours were not a problem at all. What was a problem was that she was obsessed with food, which was hurting her concentration. Given that fact that employees could eat for free at the company's cafeteria, she was concerned. Her high pressure job had begun to affect her sleep. When she took sleeping pills to get more rest, her weight crept up. She had gone from 118 to 132 pounds, and her BMI increased from 22.7 to 23.5. Though her BMI was 23.5, she saw what could be in her future if she didn't do something about it now. At thirty-three, Kate was eating a college kid's high-sugar and high-fat diet and knew that had to change. The cafeteria did offer health-conscious food. She agreed to eat more vegetables and lean protein and to eat carbs at the end of a meal.

She changed her diet and started to use the gym at work. She took advantage of the standing desks available at the office. When Kate started taking the Wellbutrin I prescribed, her obsessive thoughts about food went away. She felt more relaxed not thinking about food.

And then the marketing kicked in. Seductive and pervasive food marketing encouraged people to eat more and more food that had little resemblance to fresh, whole food. Cheap, energy-dense foods were readily accessible at fast-food restaurants, vending machines, mini marts, and convenience stores. Portions grew supersized. The double cheeseburger with bacon, fries, and a vat of soda became a staple. Thirty percent of American children have one fast-food meal a day. The way we eat has changed dramatically, and our caloric intake has gone through the roof.

# Remote Controls, Wheelies, and Other Labor-Saving Devices

At the same time overeating became the norm, we became more sedentary. Increased mechanization, motorization, urbanization, and computerization have seriously reduced our physical activity. Now machines do much of the hard labor. Technology has made getting things done more efficient, but at a cost. Remote controls, automatic garage door openers, motorized gardening equipment, and washer/ dryers all make life easier, but decrease the number of calories we burn throughout the day. Towns and neighborhoods have been developed without sidewalks. We drive everywhere. The drop in energy expenditure in the past several decades is evidenced by the fact that fewer than 50 percent of adults in the United States engage in recommended levels of physical activity.

Our children are more sedentary than previous generations. Budget cuts in education have resulted in less physical education in schools. Safety issues deprive kids of the experience of exploring their neighborhood alone or with friends. Now children's backpacks have wheels, so they don't have to carry their books to the bus or the car. Children today spend more time in front of the TV, on the Internet, or playing videogames than taking long bike rides or joining a pick-up game after school. Inactive children nourished on fast food and junk food are headed for obesity. Since 1980, the number of overweight children in the United States has doubled and the number of overweight adolescents has increased threefold.

**We are living in an obesogenic environment in which many fattening factors interact to promote the development of obesity.** Before examining some drivers of our current epidemic, we have to consider the genetic aspect of weight problems.

## Genes Are Only Part of the Story

Your tendency to gain weight is largely inherited. Your BMI is about 65 percent determined by your genes. Some people are prone to gain weight, just as some people are susceptible to developing heart disease, breast cancer, and other health problems. Weight gain and difficulty losing weight are not primarily psychological; the problems are biological.

Thousands of genes are involved in appetite, metabolism, and body weight. Large gene networks regulate energy balance. Studies have identified more than fifty specific locations of genes that are associated with body weight, BMI, and fat distribution. The Human Obesity Gene Map has located thirteen genes involved with body composition, twelve genes for fat distribution, four related to energy expenditure, and seven responsible for changes in body weight and body composition. There are now 135 candidate genes linked to weight gain and obesity.

Known as "thrifty" or obesity genes, each of these fat-promoting genes is probably responsible for a small percentage of your propensity to gain weight. You may not have inherited every single obesity gene, but like the two-thirds of the population of the United States who are overweight or obese, you probably inherited enough of them to raise your risk for gaining weight since before the day you were born. We know that obesity results from the interaction of genetics and environment. Your genetic background coupled with an environment that promotes weight gain—in other words, an obesogenic environment—can put you on the path to weight control problems.

Researchers at several institutions have determined that ten times as many weight-regulating genes are designed to increase body weight as to decrease it. It makes sense if you consider that survival depended on having energy stores. Genetics and physiology protected humans from starving during lean times of drought or harsh winters. Genes that prevent starvation promote obesity. Populations like the South Sea Islanders and Southwest Native Americans, who have endured periods of starvation, are more likely to be obese. Those with a tendency toward leanness died of starvation, and those who were overweight survived and passed their genes to subsequent generations. We like to say that Darwin got his familiar saying wrong: it's survival of the fattest. The fattest are the fittest in the wild environment.

Even if you have a genetic predisposition to gain weight, it is not written in stone. What you have inherited is not necessarily destiny. We are beginning to understand the mechanism, the epigenome, that turns those genes on and off. As a result, you may have genes for obesity that never get activated. The new science of epigenetics studies the influence of the environment and behavior on genetic expression.

Epigenetics means "above" or "on top of" the genome, as the complete set of DNA in a cell is called. The epigenome consists of chemical compounds that modify, or mark, the genome in a way that tells it what to do, where to do it, and when to do it. Although the marks are not part of the DNA itself, they can be passed on from cell to cell as cells divide and from one generation to the next. Epigenetic modifications happen when chemical alterations act as a genetic on/off switch for the DNA you have inherited. In other words, the epigenome is where the genome and the environment intersect. Your lifestyle can expose you to chemicals that change your epigenome, including what you eat and drink, the medicine you take, and the pollutants to which you are exposed.

DNA methylation is a type of mark that directly affects DNA. With methylation, chemical tags known as methyl groups attach to the DNA molecule. The methyl groups turn genes off or on by affecting interactions between DNA and a cell's protein-making machinery.

A classic experiment demonstrating how a mother mouse's diet can shape the epigenetics of her offspring illustrates how epigenetics works. The Agouti gene is present in all mammals. When the Agouti gene is methylated, as in normal mice, the expression of the gene is suppressed, the coat is brown, and the animal is protected from obesity and its complication. If the Agouti gene is unmethylated in mice, certain genes are turned on, producing offspring with yellow coats prone to obesity, diabetes, and cancer. Methyl groups come from B vitamins like folate and vitamin B12. So both fat yellow mice and skinny brown mice are genetically identical. What's the difference? When researchers fed pregnant yellow mice a methyl-rich diet, most of the next generation was brown and stayed healthy. If fed a diet deficient in B vitamins, they were yellow and obese. As you can see, epigenetic mechanisms can be boosted or impaired by the mother's diet. The results of this study show that the environment in the womb influences adult health in mice. The study provides a graphic picture of how your health is determined not only by what you eat but what your parents ate. Your mother's diet during pregnancy and your diet as an infant can affect your epigenome into adulthood.

Diets high in methyl-donating nutrients can rapidly alter gene expression, particularly during early development when the epigenome is first being established. A diet with too few methyl-donating nutrients such as folic acid or B vitamins before or after birth can cause certain regions of your DNA to be underregulated for life. A methyl-deficient diet in adulthood can lead to a decrease in DNA methylation, which can be reversed through diet. The role of nutrition during adulthood in modulating the epigenetic pattern is unclear at this point, but even so, it is interesting to know some of the nutrients believed to affect the epigenome and their sources. These nutrients have not yet been linked to obesity genes, but diets high in these methyl-donating nutrients have been shown to alter gene expression.

| Nutrient | Food Origin |
| --- | --- |
| Betaine | Wheat, spinach, shellfish, sugar beets |
| Choline | Egg yolks, liver, soy, cooked beef, chicken, veal, and turkey |
| Diallyl sulphide (DADS) | Garlic |
| Folic acid | Leafy vegetables, sunflower seeds, baker's yeast, liver |
| Methionine | Sesame seeds, Brazil nuts, fish, peppers, spinach |
| Resveratrol | Red wine |
| Sulforaphane | Broccoli |
| Vitamin B6 | Meat, whole-grain products, vegetables, nuts |
| Vitamin B12 | Meat, liver, shellfish, milk |

As you have probably noticed, most of the foods in the chart are part of a healthy, balanced diet, and very few have been processed. The takeaway? **Eating whole, fresh food is good for your epigenome.**

Epigenetics is a rich field of study that can provide us with a deeper understanding of obesity. In the future, we will be able to target weight-regulation genes and modify them through epigenetics. Epigenetic research on obesity can advance our knowledge of the mechanics of weight regulation and how to manipulate epigenetic mechanisms to combat and reverse the tendency to gain weight.

For now, the only way to manipulate epigenetics to combat obesity and weight gain is through dietary means. It is exciting to consider that breakthroughs are bound to happen in the future. In the meantime, we have to use what we know now to get the results we want.

# Six Fattening Factors Driving the Obesity Epidemic

Although much attention has been focused on the role of increased food consumption and reduced energy expenditure to explain why two-thirds of American adults are overweight, studies are showing that there are many other fattening factors in modern life that are catalysts for increased weight, some of which you would never suspect. Let's look at a few:

- Insufficient sleep

- Medications

- Endocrine disruptors or obesogens

- Air conditioning

- Social networks

- Infections

Julie had undergone a mastectomy when she was fifty-two. The stress of dealing with the surgery and taking Arimidex, the estrogen blocker medication she was taking post-surgery, caused her to put on weight in the two years after the mastectomy. She had also been taking Prozac, which may also have contributed to the change. When she came to the Comprehensive Weight Control Center, she weighed 153 pounds and was five feet tall. Her BMI was 25.5 and her waist was thirty-eight inches. She found that she was eating more desserts and drinking more alcohol. She had never had weight control problems before her surgery and was not about to be passive about gaining weight now.

We decided that she should focus on eating lower glycemic food and more protein. By focusing on lifestyle changes, July was down to 138 pounds in a year, a loss of eighteen pounds. Then she lost another seven and has maintained her weight at 131 pounds. She has lost 16 percent of her body weight.

I've chosen these because they are unexpected and interesting, but this list only scratches the surface. Other considerations include changes in distribution of ethnicity and race in the United States and the increased age of mothers when they first give birth. The effect of any one fattening factor may be small, but the combined effects of a number of factors could be significant. I have made a point to give you a sense of the number of people affected by these factors and how much things have changed in the past few decades. The rise in obesity rates parallels the rise in these statistics.

## YOU NEED TO REBOOT YOUR BODY EVERY DAY

Sleep deprivation seems to be a fact of modern life. From the glow of electronic screens to jet lag to shift work, many things interfere with getting good sleep. For example, the number of shows you've saved in your DVR queue is growing, and you have to watch them sometime. There never seem to be enough hours in the day. The average amount of sleep has steadily decreased among adults and children in the United States during the past several decades. More than 28 percent of adults in this country report that they get less than six hours of sleep a night, and this sleep debt has built up in the past three decades. Obviously, if you are awake longer, you have more opportunity to eat, and you are more likely to raid the refrigerator late at night. But sleep deprivation affects you in more profound ways. If you are not getting enough good-quality sleep, your metabolism does not function properly. Too little sleep is known to increase the risk for heart disease and to diminish mental function. Researchers are finding that even short-term, partial sleep deprivation could lead to weight gain. Studies have shown that people who had only four to six hours of sleep on consecutive nights suffered negative effects on appetite hormone signaling, eating behavior, physical activity, and rate of fat loss.

Some studies have shown that the hours of sleep you get per night are negatively correlated with BMI, meaning the more sleep you get—up to a point—the lower your BMI, and the less sleep you get, the higher your BMI, particularly in younger age groups. Studies have shown that sleep-deprived dieters lose more muscle and gain more fat than dieters who get enough rest. The amount of sleep you need does change with age, as the relationship between sleep and weight tends to taper off. Individual sleep requirements vary, so the chart that follows consists of broad recommendations.

| Age | Recommended Hours of Sleep |
| --- | --- |
| Newborns | 16 to 18 hours a day |
| Preschool-age children | 11 to 12 hours a day |
| School-age children | At least 10 hours a day |
| Teenagers | 9 to 10 hours a day |
| Adults (including the elderly) | 7 to 8 hours a day |

Leptin and ghrelin are hormones associated with appetite. Leptin suppresses appetite and speeds up metabolism, and ghrelin sends hunger signals. You will be reading a lot about these hormones in the following chapter. In one study, after two consecutive nights of only four hours of sleep, the blood levels of the hunger hormone ghrelin rose 28 percent, while levels of leptin dropped 18 percent. This change in hormone levels was accompanied by cravings for energy dense, high-carbohydrate foods and increased fat and saturated fat intake. A study of a group of women, whose sleep was reduced from seven hours to four over the course of four nights, ate an average of 400 more calories a day than they had at the start of the study. Their impulse control and their ability to delay gratification diminished with sleep deprivation, and they gained weight during the four-day study.

Depriving people of sleep for even one night has been seen to change the way their brains responded to high-calorie junk food. Fattening foods like potato chips and sweets stimulated stronger responses in the amygdala, the part of the brain that helps to control the motivation to eat. Intense activity in the almond-sized amygdala, the seat of emotions and desire in the brain, means you will eat more. At the same time, sleep deprivation has been observed to reduce activity in the frontal cortex, where higher level functions occur, including the ability to evaluate consequences and make rational decisions. This is a double whammy. **A sleep-deprived brain appears to respond more strongly to junk food and has decreased ability to curb the impulse to indulge.**

If you are not getting enough sleep, the level of the stress hormone cortisol rises, perhaps in response to inflammation. Elevated cortisol can make your body store more fat and use other tissue, like muscle, for energy. Cortisol levels naturally fall at the end of the day, so that you are able to relax and go to sleep. After getting too little sleep, people in several studies had higher levels of cortisol later in the day, which perpetuates sleep problems.

Sleep deprivation also impairs the ability of fat cells to respond to insulin. One study of young, healthy people revealed that after only four nights of reduced sleep, overall insulin sensitivity was 16 percent lower than after nights with normal sleep, and the insulin sensitivity of fat cells dropped by 30 percent. The sleep-deprived fat cells required three times as much insulin to activate the enzyme Akt,

Tom, a successful litigator, was tired all the time. He felt as if he was in a mental fog, definitely a problem for a trial lawyer. He worked relentlessly. Lately, he had no stamina and was having trouble focusing. At 6 feet 2 inches, he weighed 335 pounds, had a BMI of 42, and a waist circumference of fifty-six inches. He was fifty-seven years old and was beginning to worry that he was past his prime and getting old. He told me that he fell asleep reading every night and woke up with a headache. He was hungry all the time.

I suspected he was suffering from sleep apnea and suggested he have a sleep test. When the tests confirmed my suspicions, he agreed to sleep with a CPAP (continuous positive airway pressure) machine to correct his sleep deprivation.

He was finally able to get a good night's sleep. He was sleeping more deeply and more oxygen was circulating throughout his body to restore it after his long, intense days. He felt a surge of energy almost immediately. He had forgotten how it felt to be refreshed upon waking.

His blood tests revealed that he was insulin resistant. I prescribed metformin, a diabetes medication that can help with weight loss. His ravenous hunger diminished. He went on the Change Your Biology Diet, kept a food log, counted calories, and began to exercise. From January to June, he went from 335 to 311 pounds. That's a bit more than 7 percent of his body weight in five months. He feels as if he has been given a second chance. His renewed vitality is his greatest motivation to stay on plan to reach his weight goal—a 10 to 15 percent loss of thirty-five to fifty-two pounds.

which plays an important role in regulating blood sugar. If sleep deprivation is persistent, excess sugar and cholesterol accumulates in the bloodstream, which can lead to diabetes and heart disease. From just four nights of not getting enough sleep, the young subjects showed a ten- to twenty-year increase in metabolic age, which is calculated by comparing a person's basal metabolic rate to the basal metabolic rate of his age group, at the level of people who are obese or have diabetes.

When you are sleep deprived, you can find yourself too tired to exercise and end up using less energy. A study showed that two consecutive nights of just four hours of sleep significantly lowered the activity of subjects compared to those who slept eight hours. As you probably know, if you are not well rested, you are more lethargic. It's hard to rally to exercise if you're exhausted.

The lack of sleep disrupts the neural function of your brain cells. Adenosine is a metabolic product that builds up during the day and promotes sleepiness. Caffeine blocks the effects of adenosine, which is why a cup of coffee is a pick-me-up. Adenosine is cleared from your system when you sleep. If you do not have adequate rest, the build-up of adenosine can disrupt communication between networks in your brain. Your brain can function optimally for sixteen or seventeen hours before it needs to rest and reboot. You know what happens when you need to reboot your sluggish computer to bring it up to speed. You owe your body the rest it needs to refresh itself and restore balance.

If you average five hours of sleep a night and you start to sleep for seven or eight hours, it may be easier to lose weight. If you can reduce your sleep debt and get high-quality sleep, you will boost your metabolism and give your body the time it needs to restore itself.

## MEDICATIONS WITH FATTENING SIDE EFFECTS

The number of pharmaceuticals that have been introduced and prescribed has increased dramatically in the past three decades, paralleling the expansion of our waistlines. **Many commonly prescribed medications are known to cause weight gain. In fact, 10 percent of all obesity is caused by medications.** Some of the drugs used to treat obesity-linked conditions, such as diabetes, high blood pressure, and depression, can themselves cause weight gain.

If you are taking any medication thought to cause weight gain, you might be tempted to discontinue it in the hope of dropping pounds. That is a terrible idea.

Do not stop taking any medication without speaking to your doctor. Your doctor has prescribed the medicine for a reason, and it is important to continue taking it for your good health. If you have a prescription for a medication that causes weight gain, you and your physician can discuss finding a weight-neutral substitute. Stopping some medications abruptly can have serious side effects. Your health care provider will know the best way for you to taper off slowly and to introduce a new drug if that is possible.

Some categories of drugs that induce weight gain are:

- Antihistamines

- Diabetic

- High blood pressure

- Corticosteroids

- Antidepressants and SSRIs

- Antiseizure and mood stabilizers

- Antipsychotics

Let's take a look at the drugs that can contribute to weight gain.

### ANTIHISTAMINES

The prevalence of allergic diseases in the industrialized world has been rising for more than fifty years. The ragweed pollen season has increased by four weeks in the past ten to fifteen years, likely the result of global warming. Allergies rank fifth on the list of the leading chronic diseases in the United States. One in five people have either allergy or asthma symptoms in this country. Roughly 13 percent of people age eighteen and over in the United States have sinusitis. Worldwide, allergic rhinitis affects 10 to 30 percent of the population. These numbers mean millions of people depend on antihistamines to function for at least part of the year.

**Allergies and weight gain seem to be connected.** One study found that people who take antihistamines regularly were heavier than people who did not take them at all. Regular users were 55 percent more likely to be overweight than those not taking the drug. Regular antihistamine users weigh more, have greater BMIs and waist circumferences, and higher insulin levels. The effect appears to be more pronounced in men. When people take antihistamines like Benadryl (diphenhydramine) every day for years, they can gain weight. We often recommend newer antihistamines such as Claritin, Allegra, and Zyrtec, which are not as bad.

Histamine is a neurotransmitter that overreacts when an allergic person comes in contact with an allergen. This neurotransmitter is believed to have a secondary role in regulating appetite. In animal studies, if mice are dosed with histamine, their food intake is reduced, while antihistamines increase their appetites. Blocking histamine can disrupt an enzyme in the brain that helps to regulate food consumption. **Taking antihistamines every day for an extended period of time might affect your appetite center, causing you to eat more.**

This could be a "which came first, the chicken or the egg?" question. The situation can be viewed another way—does obesity predispose people to allergies? Obese children are more likely to suffer from allergies than children of normal weight. Inflammation could play a role. Fat cells release cytokines, chemicals that promote inflammation. If you have a greater fat mass, you may produce an exaggerated response to allergens. If your body has high levels of inflammation, you are more likely to suffer from allergies and complications like asthma. Antihistamines like diphenhydramine are the key component in most over-the-counter sleep remedies as well.

Taking them chronically for years can play a role in weight gain. We find that taking two 25 mg tablets or more is much more likely to have this effect. Melatonin, on the other hand, does not seem to cause an increase in weight, so we recommend it as an alternative.

### ANTIDEPRESSANTS AND SSRIS

During the past two decades, the use of antidepressants has sky-rocketed. After antibiotics, antidepressants are the second most prescribed drug in the United States. One in ten Americans takes medication for depression. For women in their forties and fifties, the number is one in four.

**Several antidepressants have been linked to weight gain.** The older TCAs (tricyclic antidepressants) like Elavil and Pamelor affect neurotransmitters such as serotonin, dopamine, and acetylcholine, involved in energy and appetite, and have an antihistamine effect that boosts appetite. Though SSRIs (selective serotonin reuptake inhibitors), a newer class of antidepressants like Zoloft and Prozac, are not as often linked to weight gain, Paxil appears to contribute to the highest weight increase of any of the SSRIs. Prozac and Zoloft have been associated with weight loss for the first six months, but over the long term, patients can develop a tolerance to the appetite-suppressing effect and can begin to put on weight. There are few alternatives if weight gain is an issue. Bupropion (Wellbutrin), which can generate weight loss as you will learn later, is the only antidepressant that consistently causes weight loss. Others including Remeron, Effexor, and Cymbalta, which have been considered "weight neutral," actually cause very significant weight gain in some people. **A lack of fullness is one of the complaints we heard from people taking these drugs.**

### BLOOD PRESSURE MEDICATIONS:
### BETA-BLOCKERS

Hypertension is often caused by being too heavy. One-third of American adults have high blood pressure. From the ages of fifty-five to seventy-four, that percentage goes up to half, and three-quarters of the population over seventy-five has hypertension. Taking some medication meant to lower blood pressure can cause you to put on even more weight. Beta-blockers slow down the contractions of muscle, including the skeletal muscle that burns calories. Beta-blockers, including Lopressor, Inderal, and Tenormin have been linked to weight gain. Fatigue can be a side effect of the older beta-blocker drugs. The lack of energy can lead to burning fewer calories each day. Newer beta-blockers, like Bystolic and Coreg, are less likely to cause weight gain. Calcium channel blockers, ACE (angiotensin-converting enzyme) inhibitors, and ARBs (angiotensin receptor blockers) cause little or no weight gain. We generally recommend ACE inhibitors and ARBs because they have been associated with improvement of some aspects of metabolic syndrome. Calcium channel blockers include Norvasc, Caduel, Lotrel, Exforg. Among the most commonly prescribed ACE inhibitors are Lotensin, Capoten, Vasotec, and Monopril. ARBs include Atacand, Avapro, Benicar, Cozaar, and Diovan. Several other types of blood pressure medications have also been shown to cause weight gain.

## DIABETES MEDICATION

Type 2 diabetes, an obesity-related disease, is growing worldwide. In the United States, more than one in every ten people over twenty years old has diabetes, and that figure rises to more than one in four in seniors over sixty-five. The International Diabetes Federation reported in 2013 that the global figure for people living with type 2 diabetes had surpassed 382 million. I include these figures to give you a sense of the number of people who should be taking drugs to manage their type 2 diabetes. **Unfortunately, some diabetes drugs can contribute to weight gain.**

The sulfonylurea class of diabetes medication, including DiaBeta, Glucotrol, Glipizide, and Amaryl, stimulate insulin production, which lowers blood sugar and increases appetite. Actos and Avandia, which are classed as thiazolidinediones, often increase appetite and can promote fluid retention. Metformin, the injectable GLP-1 agonists Victoza, Byetta, Bydureon, and Trulicity, and the amylin analog Symlin, are associated with weight loss. A new class of medications called SGLT-2 inhibitors, including Invokana, Farxiga, and Jardiance, can also stimulate weight loss by eliminating sugar through the kidneys.

Injected insulin itself can be associated with an increase in weight gain. In fact, in patients with little or no insulin, it is critical for restoring muscle and body fat stores. But most people with diabetes are resistant to its effects, and the use of insulin can be associated with significant weight gain. In our experience, rapid- and short-acting insulins like Humalog, Novalog, and Apidra are often associated with more weight gain than long-acting insulins like Levimir and Lantus.

### ORAL CORTICOSTEROIDS

Most corticosteroids, which are anti-inflammatory drugs, are synthetic forms of the hormone cortisone. Prednisone (Deltasone and Sterapred), methylprednisolone (Medrol), hydrocortisone (Acticort and Cortef), and dexamethasone (Decadron and Hexadrol) taken orally can carry a risk of weight gain with high dosage or long-term use. Oral corticosteroids are often prescribed for severe asthma, painful inflammatory conditions like arthritis, and many cancers. Steroids can affect your metabolic rate, can lead to increased appetite and overeating, and can promote fat storage around your middle, face, and the back of your neck. In general, steroids are only used when necessary, and strategies to prevent the weight gain need to be implemented.

### ANTISEIZURE MEDICATIONS

Some medications initially approved for the treatment of seizures are used for other purposes, including migraine headaches and mood stabilization. Valproic acid (Depakote and Depakene) is used to treat all three and can cause significant weight gain. Other medications in the category include Tegretol, Neurontin, and Lyrica, which is most often used for pain relief. Two other medications for seizures, Topamax and Zonegran, can cause significant weight loss. Studies have shown that when prescribed along with one of the weight gain–causing medicines for seizures, they can neutralize the weight gain or produce weight loss.

## ANTIPSYCHOTICS AND MOOD DISORDER

Under no circumstances should you stop or change any medication without speaking to your doctor.

Lithium, a mood stabilizer for treating bipolar disorder, is associated with weight gain, but less so than Depakote.

The mood-stabilizing atypical antipsychotic medications for bipolar disorder like clozapine (Clozaril), olanzapine (Zyprexa), risperidone (Risperdal), and quetiapine (Seroquel) have been linked to significant weight gain and diabetes. Aripiprazole (Abilify) may be better, but some people can gain a significant amount of weight. Ziprasidone (Geodon) and lurasidone (Latuda) are possible alternatives that are less likely to cause weight gain, and in some cases weight loss has been observed. These medications are often taken at night, and we sometimes see patients get ravenously hungry just before bed or wake up in the middle of the night to eat.

• • •

As you can see, the medications you take can affect your appetite and metabolism. **If you are experiencing "weight loss resistance," you might want to review the medications you are taking with your physician.** Though I've mentioned some medications as examples of weight-neutral drugs, there are many more, and pharmaceutical companies are developing new, more effective drugs without weight gain side effects.

Ted, at twenty-three, carried 299 pounds on his 6 foot 2 inch frame. He had been struggling with his weight. He had high cholesterol, sleep apnea, and fatty liver disease. The atypical antipsychotic he was taking, olanzapine, could have contributed to his weight gain. When his doctor decreased some of his medications, Ted lost twenty pounds. Then he hit a plateau.

He came to see us at 279 pounds. Even though he ate a diet high in carbs, junk food between meals, and was not physically active, Ted had managed to lose that twenty pounds. He agreed to try a low-glycemic diet. He discussed my suggestion that he begin metformin with his psychiatrist. With his doctor's go ahead, Ted starting taking metformin and lost nine pounds in three weeks. This was all the encouragement he needed.

He cut out the junk food and made certain to have a high-protein breakfast each day. He lost twenty-two pounds in three months. He got a step counter and started moving more. Ted applied to graduate school and is ready to turn his life around. Even though he was taking medication that promoted weight gain, he was able to drop pounds.

## THE COMFORT ZONE

Or as we scientists say "reduction in the variability of ambient temperature." Most of us live in a temperature-controlled environment. Though you might never have given a thought to the link between where your thermostat is set and your weight, temperature does affect how many calories you burn. Exposure to cold temperatures, which produces shivering, and high temperatures, which causes you to perspire, uses extra energy as your body works to stabilize its inner temperature. When external conditions affect your body temperature, your body will work hard to return to normal.

Your body responds quickly to heat loss from cold external temperatures. Your muscles move and twitch, causing you to shiver, which increases heat production by as much as five times its normal level. If you walk outside in frigid weather, your basal metabolic rate increases to compensate for heat loss. You end up burning more calories. A temperature-controlled environment in the cold winter months reduces the number of calories you would burn to stay warm.

Being cold also activates brown fat. We have two types of fat tissue—white and brown. White fat stores glucose and produces hormones. Brown fat contains mitochondria, organelles that are factories that burn up calories to create heat. In some ways it acts more like muscle tissue, from which it is derived, than white fat. Being cold activates brown fat, which extracts fat from the rest of the body to create heat, reducing deposits of white fat. Scientists have found that lean people tend to have more brown fat than overweight people. A temperature-controlled environment in the cold winter months keeps your brown fat dormant and reduces the number of calories you would burn to stay warm.

When the external temperature is high, your appetite is likely to be suppressed. Eating and digesting food require a lot of energy and will produce heat at a time when your body needs to stay cool or more specifically maintain a normal temperature. Thermoregulation takes precedence over appetite. In other words, it is more important to your body to control its temperature than it is to eat. When you are exposed to air-conditioned environments during the summer, you interfere with your body's natural tendency to suppress your appetite.

If you are exposed to ambient temperatures above or below the thermoneutral zone (TNZ), a range of temperatures in which expending energy is not needed to stabilize inner temperature, you will burn fat for energy. Living in a TNZ, as we do so much of the time today, contributes to fat development. Industrial livestock operations use this knowledge to set the environment to fatten up the animals, maximizing weight gain. The same thing is inadvertently happening to the population of industrialized nations. We go from our homes to our cars to our offices, malls, gyms, and theaters where the environment is comfort controlled. Compared to decades ago, we spend a lot more time in the TNZ. In the winter, we've turned up the temperature indoors. In 1926, the thermal standard for winter comfort in the United States was 64.4°F. That number had risen to 76.3 by 1986. Between 1978 and 1997, homes in the United States with central air conditioning rose from 23 to 47 percent. The latest results from the 2009 Residential Energy Consumption Survey show that

87 percent of households in the United States are equipped with air conditioning. Though we may live in comfort, this aspect of modern life has a role in making ours an overweight society.

A more variable indoor temperature, which rises and falls with the temperature outside, could prove to be beneficial. A Japanese research group found a decrease in body fat after people spent two hours a day at 62.6°F for six weeks. Up to middle age, nonshivering heat production can account for up to 30 percent of a body's energy budget. Lower temperatures can significantly affect the overall amount of energy you expend. **With this in mind, lowering your thermostat in the winter and getting out in the cold to take a walk can stimulate your metabolism.** Allow yourself to be hot enough to perspire a bit in the summer, and you may want to eat less.

OBESOGENS

The hormones in your body are chemical messengers that communicate among your organs, your brain, and the environment. There is a class of synthetic chemicals called endocrine disruptors that interfere with the production of hormones and how they do their jobs. These chemicals can trick your body in many ways. They can increase the production of certain hormones and decrease the production of others. Some endocrine disruptors mimic hormones, particularly estrogen, while others have the power to turn one hormone into another. Endocrine disruptors may turn on, turn off, or modify the signals that hormones carry, which may affect the normal functions of tissues and organs. Even low doses of these chemicals may have negative effects. Exposure to endocrine disruptors can cause genetic and epigenetic changes that are passed to future generations.

In the past decade, evidence has been mounting that suggests certain of these endocrine disruptors may be playing a role in the obesity epidemic. These chemicals have been labeled "obesogens." For some people, obesogens may be altering metabolism and fat cell development, making it harder for them to maintain a healthy weight. Obesogens interfere with the mechanisms important for weight control. BPA (bisphenol A) is such a compound, and has been shown to demethylate DNA, thus making weight gain and the development of glucose intolerance and diabetes easier.

Exposure to obesogens is especially critical early in life. A developing fetus or infant is vulnerable, because neither has the protections that are available to adults, such as a fully developed immune system, blood-brain barrier, DNA repair mechanism, and detoxifying enzymes. Research is emerging that finds exposure to certain environmental chemicals during development may play a role in becoming obese later in life. There can be a time lag between exposure and manifestation of a disease. The early stages of life are a critical time, because the number of fat cells is being programmed and metabolic set points are being established. Damage done prenatally is more likely to be irreversible than disruptions that occur in adulthood.

Weight gain associated with these chemicals tends to occur at low levels of exposure. How these chemicals cause weight gain is not yet known but may involve altered thyroid function and metabolism and energy homeostasis.

If you want to reduce your exposure to endocrine disruptors, there are a number of things you can do that are part of the Change Your Biology Diet. Aside from minimizing the amount of plastic in your life, you have to take control over what you eat. **If you eat fresh, whole food, you do not have to worry as much about what additives you are consuming.** Some people prefer to eat organic produce and meat to avoid pesticides, antibiotics, and hormones used in conventional farming.

There is no way to avoid endocrine disruptors completely. They are pervasive in modern life. At first, I was not going to write about obesogens for that reason. I didn't want you to feel overwhelmed and lose heart. But I do think it is important for you to be aware of the many external factors that influence your weight and the way your body stores energy. When you recognize that some things are beyond your control, you might have an easier time focusing on what you can do.

At this time, there are about twenty known obesogens, but the field is relatively young. Since we live in a chemical age, more endocrine disruptors that affect weight gain are bound to be discovered. BPA, phytoestrogens, phthalates, and organotins have been associated with obesity. An examination of these endocrine disruptors will give you a sense of how pervasive these chemicals are.

## BPA (BISPHENOL A)

According to government tests, 93 percent of Americans have BPA in their bodies. Used to harden plastics and epoxy resins, it is found in plastic bottles, can lining, thermal paper used for cash register receipts, polycarbonate baby bottles and other containers, and household electronics. BPA mimics estrogen and has been linked to heart disease, insulin resistance, and obesity. This hormone disruptor can stimulate the release of pro-inflammatory substances from fat tissue, which are involved in insulin resistance and metabolic syndrome. BPA has been shown to affect the epigenome by removing methyl groups from DNA. In an animal study, exposure to BPA during pregnancy is associated with obesity in male offspring. Being exposed to BPA during pregnancy mimics the effects of a high fat diet and alters blood sugar balance and gene expression in male offspring

**How to Avoid BPA:** Eat fresh rather than canned foods. Many food cans are lined with BPA. You can research companies that do not use BPA in their products. At the supermarket or home goods store, look for the label "BPA-Free." Stay away from plastics marked with a "PC," for polycarbonate or recycling label #7. Though not all of these plastics contain BPA, many do. Even cash register receipts use BPA to bind the ink to the paper. And the use of a hand sanitizer significantly increases the amount of BPA absorbed.

## PHYTOESTROGENS

Phytoestrogens, found most prominently in soybeans and soy products, are substances found in plants that have estrogen-like properties. There are two main types of phytoestrogens: isoflavones and lignans. Genistein is the most abundant isoflavone in soy. Genistein can either increase or decrease the effects of estrogen. It binds to estrogen receptors on cells and stimulates the receptors, but not as strongly as real estrogen, and blocks estrogen from attaching. Genistein is believed to regulate a healthy fat and carbohydrate balance. A recent study showed that at high doses genistein did inhibit the growth of fat tissue, but at low doses, as found in soy milk or food supplements containing soy, it increased the accumulation of fat tissue, especially in men, and promoted mild insulin resistance. Phytoestrogens, alone or in combination with other chemicals, have many pathways of action and are likely involved in energy metabolism and fat storage. As research continues, we will learn more about the role of these phytoestrogens in body weight.

**How to Avoid Phytoestrogens:** If you are having problems losing weight and are a big consumer of phytoestrogens, you might want to avoid soy products for a period of time and see what happens. You can continue to eat fermented soy products such as tempeh, miso, and natto.

## ORGANOTINS-TBT

Organotins are a class of persistent organic pollutants (POP), hazardous air pollutants, that have been present in the air we breathe since the 1950s. They are used as fungicides and pesticides on crops, as wood preservatives, in vinyl products (PVC) including toys, school supplies, floor tile, rain jackets, shower curtains, food wrap, PVC water pipes, other plastic products made from polyesters, and polyurethane foam. It is impossible to know all the uses of organotins in products you use every day, but be aware that they are hard to avoid.

TBT (tributyltin), a highly toxic organotin, has been found to disrupt normal development and controls over the development of fat cells and energy balance. TBT has been shown to cause permanent changes in mice exposed during prenatal development, resulting in a predisposition for weight gain.

**How to Avoid Organotins:** Do not use products made of polyvinyl chloride plastic. You can find lists of PVC-free products for your home. Try to minimize your use of other plastic and foam products.

## PERFLUOROOCTANOIC ACID (PFOA) AND PHTHALATES

Phthalate plasticizers, some of which are also xenoestrogens, used to soften PVC plastics, and various PFCs (perfluoro alkyl compound), used as surface repellents, can promote fat production. Prenatal exposure to low to moderate levels of PFOA in rodents led to decreased fat mass and body weight. Chronic low-level exposure to PFOA depressed birth weight, but increased fat tissue mass and weight gain after puberty.

**How to Avoid Phthalates:** Stay away from plastic food containers, children's toys, plastic wrap made from PVC, which has the recycling label #3. Some personal care products contain phthalates, including baby lotion, deodorants, and hair gels. Read the labels and avoid products that use the catch-all term "fragrance," which sometimes means hidden phthalates.

### THE SOCIAL NETWORK

Research has shown that social interactions play a role in the obesity epidemic. One of the questions is whether obesity can spread from person to person like a "contagious" disease. There is compelling research that finds the answer could be "yes." Researchers investigated 12,067 people who participated in the Framingham Heart Study. From 1971 to 2003, the subjects had many medical evaluations for the study.

They found that if one sibling became obese during the study, the chance that another sibling would become obese increased by 40 percent. In the case of siblings, genetics could have had something to do with it. If a spouse became obese, the other spouse's chances of doing the same rose by 37 percent. That increase could be explained away by shared lifestyle habits and meals. The scientists also found that if someone's friend became obese, the likelihood of his crossing the 30 BMI line was up 57 percent. They found that physical proximity was not that important with friends. Having an obese neighbor had much less influence than an obese friend, no matter how far away the friend lived. Friends of the same sex were especially influential. A man with a male friend who became obese had the greatest chance of growing obese himself. These numbers indicate that the influences of genetics and shared environment do not explain why obesity occurs in social clusters.

Though scientists do not fully understand how obesity spreads, they believe what members of a social network consider normal and acceptable is an important factor. If a man sees his friends gain weight over time, he might view the change as natural. Rather than adopting a lifestyle that would help him manage his weight, he might just resign himself and be like others he knows. In the end, people might be influenced more by others who look like them than by those who are different. Given the prevalence of obesity, people's perception of what is normal can contribute to making obesity acceptable.

# Obesity Goes Viral

During the past thirty years, nearly a dozen microbes have been linked with animal or human obesity, including viruses, bacteria, and parasites. The adenovirus 36 (Ad-36) has been of particular interest. In the late 1970s, commercial chicken growers in Mumbai, India, were troubled by deaths in their flocks. They found that the virus SMAM-1, also known as avian virus, lowered the immune system of infected chickens, which eventually killed them. In the process, the growers noticed that the body fat of the chickens increased. SMAM-1 became the first adenovirus reported to increase fat tissue. Some humans have developed antibodies to the chicken virus, meaning they had been infected. In 1978, adenovirus 36 (Ad-36) was identified. Scientists believe the human virus arose from SMAM-1.

Adenovirus 36 is linked to upper respiratory infection, conjunctivitis, and sometimes gastrointestinal symptoms. You can develop this viral infection if you are exposed to droplets from the coughs or sneezes of an infected person. The virus stays alive for one to two months, and others can be infected during that time.

The human adenovirus was found in studies to increase fat storage in animals. Experiments on chickens, mice, and rats showed up to three times greater weight gain and 60 percent increase in fat tissue in Ad-36 infected animals as opposed to animals that were not infected. Ad-36 infected monkeys studied over a period of seven months gained four times as much weight and increased their body fat by 60 percent more than the control group. Since the virus promotes fat growth and weight gain by increasing glucose and lipid uptake in cells, it lowers cholesterol and triglycerides in the bloodstream. An Ad-36 infection was associated with a 15 percent increase in body weight and a 29 percent drop in cholesterol levels in rhesus monkeys.

Many studies have been done that show that people who test positive for Ad-36 are more prone to gain weight and become obese than those who have never encountered the virus. A study of 1,400 people who tested positive for antibodies to the virus, revealing that they had been infected at some point, gained more fat over a ten-year period than noninfected people, but the infected people had lower blood sugar. Among 500 adults in three U.S. cities, 30 percent of obese adults had been infected by Ad-36, but only 11 percent of people of normal weight had been. Those who had been infected had a BMI on average nine units heavier than noninfected people. The weight effects of Ad-36 are especially evident in children. Twenty-two to 30 percent of obese children have been infected, while only 7 to 14 percent of non-obese children have.

Ad-36 causes chronic changes in the biochemistry and physiology of the person who has the virus. When the virus invades the cells of the lining of the blood vessels in the upper respiratory region, its DNA enters the cells and migrates to the nucleus to replicate. The host cells die and release viral particles into the blood where they infect other tissue. Ad-36 seems to reach the brain, lung, liver, and fat tissue very quickly. The viral DNA turns on transcription factors, proteins that determine which genes are turned on or off, and enzymes that produce obesity. The virus prompts adult stem cells, which are undifferentiated cells, to convert to specialized fat cells in adipose tissue, producing more fat cells. Fat tissue from an infected animal has bigger fat cells, and more of them, than an animal who has not been infected. The virus also triggers an increase of glucose receptors in cell membranes, which enables cells to take in increased levels of glucose. At the same time, the virus increases the production of the enzyme that converts glucose into fatty acids, increasing the fat within the fat cells. This might be why blood lipid levels go down in people who have been infected. Ad-36 also lowers the amount of the appetite-suppressing hormone leptin produced by fat cells. This is a perfect storm for weight gain and alteration of body composition.

·  ·  ·

All these fattening factors, drivers of obesity, have come on the scene in the past fifty years or so and parallel the steady rise in obesity we have been seeing. Think of your body as a big stockpot of simmering soup on the stovetop. As you add one ingredient after another and turn up the heat, the soup eventually boils over. There are so many things in our obesogenic environment that affect the energy balance in the body. A combination of many factors can put you over the top.

**Now you have an idea of the many external factors that contribute to weight gain.** The next chapter focuses on what goes on in your body that causes an expanding waistline and increased weight. Research has found that eating too much high-calorie food changes your brain and damages the nerves in your appetite control center.

# CHAPTER 3

# Why Don't People Just Lose Weight?

SO FAR, WE'VE HAD A LOOK at many of the external factors that trigger weight gain. I opened this book by referring to mechanisms in your body that can make losing weight difficult. We have made important breakthroughs in understanding in this area of research. This chapter focuses on the physical processes inside your body that cause you to put on weight and make losing those excess pounds a challenge. This is a ratcheting phenomenon. When you eat too much and don't exercise, you gain weight that you can't seem to take off. You are fighting against a real resistance in your body.

## It Is Your Hormones, After All — At Least in Part

In the past, it was common to assume that thyroid hormone imbalance was at the root of weight gain, because the hormone plays a key role in regulating metabolism. Yet when patients with weight problems are given thyroid medication, they do not necessarily lose weight. The use of thyroid hormone to treat obesity has proven not to be as useful as some thought it would be, because the relationship among metabolic rates, energy balance, and weight change is very complex. Thyroid hormone alone is not the answer. There are many other hormones, proteins, and chemicals that have significant effects on your ability to manage your weight. All these substances interact with the brain centers that regulate energy expenditure, appetite, and storage of unburned energy as fat.

## INSULIN RESISTANCE

Up to 75 percent of Americans are insulin resistant and unaware that they are in this prediabetic condition. Some symptoms ascribed to insulin resistance might be familiar to you, but these are not specific enough to diagnose insulin resistance:

- Trouble losing weight

- Extra fat around the middle and a high fat to lean tissue ratio

- Cravings for sweet and/or salty snacks

- Carbohydrate addiction

- Afternoon fatigue

- Brain fog

- Sleepiness and bloating after a high-carb meal

- Agitation, mood swings, nausea, or headaches that are rapidly relieved once food is eaten

- Depression

Insulin is a hormone that regulates carbohydrate and fat metabolism and plays a significant role in weight gain. Insulin sends messages to brain cells to order cells to process blood sugar for energy and to signal that no more food is needed. When your body is properly sensitive to the hormone insulin, it signals for the cells to absorb glucose from the bloodstream.

The food you eat, composed of fat, protein, carbohydrates, vitamins, and minerals, is digested and broken down to smaller

Sean, a chef, wanted to lose weight but wasn't willing to change what he ate. After all, he reasoned, food was what he did for a living. He was on his feet all day in the kitchen, but he never got any other exercise. In addition, he worked late until the restaurant closed, and he wasn't getting enough sleep. At five feet six inches, he weighed 237 pounds and had a BMI of 38.2. He was taking Actos for his diabetes, a medication that can lead to weight gain. I switched him from Actos to Invokana. I added metformin to his medications. He began to lose weight steadily. After three months, he had lost fourteen pounds. He was eating less than he used to, but still eating more than he should if he wanted to keep losing. I added Victoza to speed the weight loss process.

After six months, he was down to 207 pounds, a loss of 12.7 percent of his body weight in nine months. Sean did make an effort to eat less and cut down on bread and soda. He even started having a protein shake for breakfast. He was still craving carbohydrates and began to eat more junk food. I added bupropion to help him to control the cravings, and he continued to lose during the next four months. He got down to 182, and his BMI was 29.4. I retested his blood glucose and found that Sean had hit the normal range in both the fasting blood sugar test and the long-term A1C test that compares blood sugar levels over a three-month period. With his diabetes under control, losing weight was going to be easier for him.

Sean was so encouraged, he added high-intensity exercise to the mix and managed to change what he ate without interfering with his work. He claims he has become a more creative chef because of his new take on healthy food.

components that are more easily absorbed by the body. The proteins and nutrients are used for cellular metabolism, immune function, and cell replacement. When carbohydrates are broken down, they produce glucose, your body's basic fuel, which, in the form of blood sugar, is carried in the bloodstream to the cells. Just as your brain needs oxygen, it needs stable blood sugar levels to function well. Insulin, which is produced by the pancreas, signals the cells to absorb glucose from the bloodstream for energy and regulates how much glucose remains in the bloodstream. As blood glucose levels rise after a meal, the pancreas releases insulin to help cells absorb and use the glucose.

When you gain weight, the metabolism of your fat cells changes. Their ability to receive the insulin signal into the cell becomes compromised. Since the cells' ability to respond to insulin is diminished, more insulin is needed to enable glucose to enter. The pancreas produces more insulin to meet the increased demand. Elevated insulin levels can cause cells to ignore the messages, a condition called insulin resistance. With insulin resistance, the body does not use insulin properly, and muscle and liver cells do not respond to the signals from insulin. But fat cells do respond, and as a result store more calories away as fat.

The more simple carbohydrates you eat, the more insulin your pancreas produces. Eating sweets and refined starches, which are rapidly digested, causes blood sugar levels to spike, which exaggerates the insulin response. Eventually, the pancreas can't keep up with the need for insulin, and glucose builds up in the bloodstream, setting the stage for diabetes. When blood glucose levels begin to rise higher than normal, you are in a prediabetic state.

If insulin levels remain too high, cells in the body and brain stop responding. The message doesn't get through that there is too much energy in the body. Muscle cells stop burning as much fuel, your metabolism slows, and less blood sugar is used for energy. Insulin triggers the liver to convert excess sugar in the bloodstream to triglycerides, which are stored in your fat cells and contribute to even greater insulin resistance. Insulin resistance is most often associated with high triglycerides.

**If you are insulin resistant and eat simple carbohydrates, you need up to five times the amount of insulin to bring your blood glucose to healthy levels.** When insulin spikes because of high glucose levels, the glucose is stored in fat cells. The more fat you have, the more insulin resistant you become. The complications that result from insulin resistance are referred to as CHAOS, which stands for:

- C—Coronary artery disease

- H—Hypertension

- A—Adult onset diabetes (type 2)

- O—Obesity

- S—Stroke

The good news is that you can improve or even correct this condition by means of diet and exercise. Lowering the amount of insulin your pancreas needs to produce can help you to reduce fat and lose weight. If you eat a diet high in sugar and simple carbohydrates, like white bread and potatoes, which quickly break down to glucose, your body will need more insulin to deal with all the blood glucose that is circulating. A typical American diet, consisting of supersized fast foods, sodas, and sweets, is a recipe for developing insulin resistance. Caffeine, artificial sweeteners, nicotine, stress, and steroid medications can also contribute to insulin resistance. In the next chapter, you will learn how to eat to keep your blood sugar level from spiking or crashing so that energy production stays on an even keel.

## FAT CELLS AS DYNAMIC ENDOCRINE ORGANS

Adipose tissue does more than serve as a source of energy. Fat cells are very active at producing chemical messages that communicate with other organs. For example, some of these hormones communicate with immune cells. As a result, excess calorie storage expands adipose tissue and initiates an inflammatory response, which is a cause of many of the complications we associate with obesity. Not only does insulin resistance lead to reduced absorption of blood glucose, but insulin no longer applies a "metabolic brake" on the release of fatty acids and hormones from fat cells. Normally, insulin binds to the insulin receptor on the surface of fat cells and inhibits the activity of HSL (hormone sensitive lipase), which limits the secretion of fatty acids. When fatty acids are released from fat cells, they activate stress hormones and inflammation. If BMI is high, excessive fat tissue can produce an acute inflammatory response that leads to chronic inflammation.

Fat cells produce more than fifty inflammatory substances, called adipokines, which affect metabolism, energy balance, and cardiovascular function. These bioactive substances include tumor necrosis factor (TNF-a), the interleukins, C-reactive protein (CRP), angiotensin, resistin, and leptin, an important regulator of food intake to be discussed in more detail later in this chapter. Excessive fat stores reduce secretion of adiponectin, an anti-inflammatory protein that enhances insulin sensitivity in the liver and muscle. As adipose tissue accumulates, production of this protein decreases. These adipokines are directly or indirectly involved in processes that lead to cardiovascular disease, hypertension, insulin resistance, type 2 diabetes, and cholesterol problems. In addition to promoting inflammation, some of these adipokines further increase insulin resistance, setting another vicious cycle into play.

Adipokines are the link between having too much body fat, metabolic syndrome, and cardiovascular disease. Numerous studies have found that obese individuals have higher pro-inflammatory cytokines and lower anti-inflammatory cytokines than healthy, lean people. The more adipose tissue you have, the more inflammatory factors are released. Inflammation begins in the fat cells themselves. As fat mass expands, inflammation increases. Obesity places stress on the cells, particularly on the mitochondria, the power plant in each cell. As more glucose is delivered to fat cells, an inflammatory cascade happens within the cell. Elevated levels of inflammatory cytokines predict future weight gain. Weight loss reduces the levels of most pro-inflammatory adipokines, alleviates inflammation, and enhances insulin sensitivity. The Change Your Biology Diet gives you a way to eat that will help you achieve these desired results.

## LEPTIN RESISTANCE

Obesity research took a giant step when leptin, a hormone produced by fat tissue, was discovered at Rockefeller University in 1994. What was riveting about this discovery was that it demonstrated that adipose tissue was able to signal the central nervous system—in other words, your fat has direct communication with your brain. I was there to observe some of the early studies. My colleague Rudy Leibel, who is now the director of the Division of Molecular Genetics in the Department of Pediatrics at Columbia, left Mass General and Harvard to study obesity at Rockefeller University. The move was precipitated when a patient walked out of his office in the early 1980s because Dr. Leibel and his colleagues had little to offer by way of weight management programs. His goal at Rockefeller was to find what drove eating and to find the connection between obesity and genetics. He collaborated with many other scientists at Rockefeller, including Yiying Zhang and Dr. Jeffrey Friedman, who are credited with discovering the gene, to initiate the research that ultimately led to the discovery of leptin.

In 1986, I was at a faculty meeting concerning the Weill Cornell medical students. Dr. Leibel sought me out because he had heard I was interested in obesity and had started a treatment program. He invited me to his lab to see what they were working on. Among a number of normal-size mice, he pointed out a very fat mouse, four or five times the size of the others. The mouse was so large it couldn't move. He believed that a gene mutation in the code for a hormone, which floats in the bloodstream as a messenger to other organs, was responsible for the weight gain. An abnormal version of the hormone was being made by the defective gene and as a result, the mouse's brain couldn't tell how much fat was stored, so it kept on storing more and more. The fat mouse became skinny in just three days when it was given a transfusion from the skinny mice. They proved that something in the blood kept mice at normal weight. That communication wasn't happening in the fat mouse I observed. Rudy began and played a key role in the research that led to the discovery of that hormone. Leptin, as we now know, activates signals in the hypothalamus, a pearl-size structure deep in your brain. Their discovery gave us a new approach to obesity, which is the basis of the Change Your Biology Diet.

Leptin is produced by fat cells. The more body fat you have, the higher your leptin levels will be. Obese people can have up to ten times more leptin in their blood as thin people. That might seem like a good thing, because there is more leptin circulating to tell the brain that you are no longer hungry. But it doesn't work that way. What happens is similar to insulin resistance. An excess of fat cells in the body produces an overload of leptin, which doesn't seem to be useful. Either leptin is not getting to your brain, or your brain is not responding to the message. Leptin receptors seem to be less sensitive to leptin's message. **You might once have felt full within just ten minutes of eating a big meal, but with excess weight these signals may take much longer to induce a feeling of fullness.** The fullness you do experience is milder than it used to be, so you are not persuaded to stop eating. Eventually, you may still feel hungry even when you've just eaten large quantities of food. You may never feel really hungry, but you also never feel full, so you graze on and on with no signals to make you stop. Your damaged neurons no longer respond to leptin, a condition called leptin resistance.

Your weight is controlled by complex interactions between hormones and nerves in the hypothalamus. If you are overweight, you can develop what I call a "feed-forward" mechanism. **Consuming too many calories from sugar and fat overloads and inflames the neurons in the hypothalamus, causing them to deteriorate prematurely and trigger inflammation.** What happens next is that pathways in the brain resist normal signals like leptin, which tell the brain how much fat is stored, and signals from the stomach and intestines, which tell the brain how much and what has been eaten. The calorie surge caused by eating too many calories of "fattening" food disrupts your appetite feedback loops. **Signals about how much fat is stored are blocked, making your brain think you need more energy.**

A diet high in saturated fat and simple carbohydrates sets off a chain reaction of metabolic dysfunction that involves the appetite-regulating hormones leptin and ghrelin. Leptin activates the appetite-suppressing pathways, so that when hormones come from the intestine and stomach, the brain can tell how much food has been eaten. Leptin doesn't make you feel full, but without it, the system

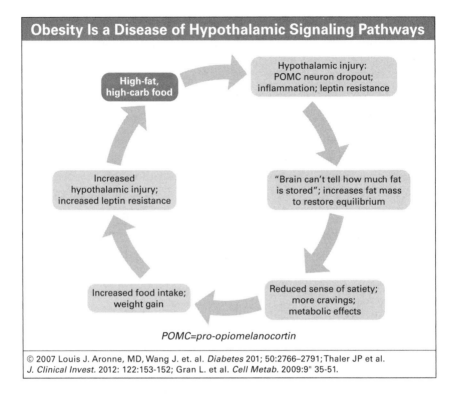

## Obesity Is a Disease of Hypothalamic Signaling Pathways

High-fat, high-carb food

Hypothalamic injury: POMC neuron dropout; inflammation; leptin resistance

"Brain can't tell how much fat is stored"; increases fat mass to restore equilibrium

Reduced sense of satiety; more cravings; metabolic effects

Increased food intake; weight gain

Increased hypothalamic injury; increased leptin resistance

POMC=pro-opiomelanocortin

© 2007 Louis J. Aronne, MD, Wang J. et. al. *Diabetes* 201; 50:2766–2791; Thaler JP et al. *J. Clinical Invest.* 2012: 122:153-152; Gran L. et al. *Cell Metab.* 2009:9" 35-51.

doesn't work properly and you don't feel full when you should. When you gain weight, your brain becomes resistant to these signals. When you lose weight, your leptin levels drop precipitously, which makes the appetite-suppressing pathways less effective, and your stomach produces a hormone called ghrelin, which increases hunger. When you're resistant to leptin or you don't have enough around, you have difficulty fighting off the increase in appetite from your stomach's production of ghrelin. In a sense, your brain has gone haywire, and you can't trust the messages it's sending you about appetite, hunger, and fullness. **I explain to my patients that it's as if their gas gauge points to empty all the time, whether or not the tank is full. They keep stopping for gas and start filling up gas cans and storing them in the trunk of their car, because they are convinced they will run out of gas at any moment.** That's how the "feed-forward" mechanism operates.

Animal research has shown that adding fat, particularly saturated fat, to the usual high-carbohydrate diet in animals bred to become obese results in very early and lasting injury to the neurocircuits in the hypothalamus that control energy and metabolism. Similar damage has been found in the same area of the brain in obese humans. The development of new neurons slows down and the remaining older neurons do not function as well. Years of eating the typical American diet actually change the brain by damaging the signaling pathways in the hypothalamus. I repeat: the overload from poor eating damages your brain.

**The evidence shows that fattening food increases the body weight set-point by impairing the production of new nerves.** Lowering this set-point appears to improve the process, at least temporarily. Though some hypothalamic injury may be permanent, some may be reversed. If you eat less high-fat, high-carbohydrate food, you appear to reduce the rate of damage. Some researchers have found that omega-3 fatty acids found in fish oil appear to modulate some of the negative effects of carbohydrates and saturated fats. Studies of mice have shown that nerve growth factor can repair "burn out" damage. Recently, researchers at Boston's Children's Hospital have discovered a unique anti-inflammatory compound that overcomes leptin resistance. Both approaches produce profound weight loss in mice. The second approach is very promising, in that it may actually be repairing the damage that occurs, allowing signaling from leptin as well as other hormones to improve. But permanent weight loss takes time. The brain's metabolic messaging system needs to heal. The Change Your Biology Diet is designed to minimize that damage and to give your brain time to repair itself. The low-carb/high-protein diet we recommend has been shown to improve neurogenesis.

## A WORD ON GHRELIN, THE HUNGER HORMONE

Discovered in 1999, ghrelin is a hormone, released from cells in the stomach, which stimulates hunger. Ghrelin sends a signal to the hypothalamus and the reward centers of the brain to urge you to eat. Ghrelin levels change dramatically during the course of a day—rising sharply before a meal and taking a dive after you eat. Ghrelin

Andy was diagnosed with cancer of the kidney. His doctors wanted him to take off forty pounds before he had surgery. At five feet eleven inches, he weighed 271 pounds and had a BMI of 37.8. His surgeons told him there would be less risk of complications if he could get his weight within a normal range. He was forty-two and wanted to deal with the cancer as soon as he could, so he made an appointment to see me.

We started with lifestyle changes. He hadn't been taking very good care of himself. In fact, he was clueless about good nutrition. He binged on a lot of junk food filled with saturated fat. Bacon cheeseburgers and fries was his go-to meal. He was sedentary. He started on the Change Your Biology Diet. Andy made certain to have a high-protein breakfast, increased his activity, and paid attention to the glycemic level of the food he ate. Having lost four pounds in two months, he was showing signs of "weight loss resistance." We agreed that he needed medication to jump-start more significant weight loss. He starting taking metformin once a day, and Belviq once a day. In six weeks' time, he had lost a total of eighteen pounds. We increased the metformin and Belviq to twice a day, and he continued to stay on plan with his eating. Within six months, he had lost forty pounds. At 231 pounds, his BMI was 22.7. He was ready for surgery, which had a great outcome.

stimulates the brain to increase appetite, slows metabolism, and decreases the ability to burn fat. Ghrelin promotes visceral fat storage.

People with obesity do not have as big a suppression in ghrelin following a meal compared to people of normal weight, a possible reason why they eat more. Gastric bypass surgery seems to fix this. Ghrelin remains elevated following weight loss, one of the many hormonal changes that contribute to weight regain.

# Why and How Your Body
# Resists Losing Weight

Earlier, we discussed the immediate health benefits of losing just 5 to 10 percent of your body weight. This improvement carries over to pro-inflammatory hormone levels, which improve significantly with just a 5 to 10 percent weight loss. Good cholesterol goes up and triglycerides and blood sugar go down. But when you lose between 5 to 10 percent of your weight, your brain reacts as if you've lost much more of your body fat, and alarms go off indicating that your energy stores have been depleted—your gas tank is emptying fast! Your body can react to weight loss by signaling how much you should weigh and pushing you back up to a set point. Losing weight is associated with changes in levels of hormones that trigger the production of neuropeptides that induce hunger and decrease energy expenditure. **With weight loss, hormones that inhibit food intake and increase energy expenditure are suppressed. In other words, you get hungry and your metabolism slows down. Your body wants to regain that weight.**

When you lose weight, leptin drops dramatically and ghrelin goes up. Everything is moving in the wrong direction! A 10 to 15 percent weight loss can reduce leptin by 50 percent. If you were two hundred pounds and lost twenty, your leptin would be down 50 percent at 180 pounds. A 10 percent weight loss also reduces your metabolism, 20 to 25 percent, and muscle metabolism 30 to 40 percent during physical activity. Several factors play a role in these changes. Your muscles become more efficient, burning fewer calories for the same amount of exercise, and thyroid, leptin, and intestinal hormone levels fall. Evidence shows that a reduction of body fat stimulates this network of overlapping neuroendocrine systems that acts to increase appetite and decrease metabolism. That is why maintaining weight loss very difficult. Though I am not going to discuss the substances that regulate energy balance in detail, I will list them, just so you know the number of hormones, neurotransmitters, and peptide hormone, produced in the brain or in places such as fat tissue, muscle, and the gastro intestinal tract, that are at play:

## Decrease Food Intake
- Leptin
- a-Melanocyte-stimulating hormone
- Corticotropin-releasing hormone

- Thryotropin-releasing hormone
- Cholecycstokinin
- Somatostatin
- Glucagon-like peptide 1
- Urocortin
- Neuromedin
- Serotonin
- Dopamine
- Acrp30/apm-1/GBP28
- C75/Cerulenin

**Increase Food Intake**
- Ghrelin
- Neuropeptide Y
- AGRP
- MCH
- Orexin/Hypocretin
- Galanin
- Norepeinephrine
- Perilipin

There are many other peptides, neurotransmitters, cytokines, steroid hormones, and enzymes that affect energy balance in your body. The complexity of our bodies never stops amazing me.

# The Gut-Brain-Gut Axis

In addition to these hormonal factors regulating metabolism and appetite, there are important signals carried by nerves as well. The vagus nerve is the main nerve of the gastrointestinal tract that helps to regulate body weight. A right and left vagus connect the GI tract to the brain. The vagus nerve runs from the brain through the esophagus and branches out to reach nearly every part of the digestive system. When the stomach is empty, the vagus nerve informs the brain and triggers the feeling of hunger. When there is food in the stomach, the vagus communicates with the brain and relays the brain's commands to secrete stomach acid to digest the food and feel full. Without the vagus, we would get less hungry and food would stay longer in the stomach.

The brain instructs the pancreas through the vagus nerve to make insulin as food is being digested and instructs fat tissues to absorb more nutrients. The vagus is essentially an energy storage nerve, designed to make you consume energy and store it in your fat.

Research has shown that obesity impairs signaling from the vagus nerve. This method of communication between the intestine and the brain becomes disrupted and does not return to normal once weight is lost. The nerves in the stomach that signal fullness to the brain appear to be desensitized after long-term consumption of a high-fat diet. In animal studies, it takes more food to induce satiety in subjects exposed to a chronic high-fat diet than it does in low-fat-fed subjects. When this happens, more food must be consumed to feel full.

As you will see in Chapter 10, one of the latest approved treatments for obesity is an electronic vagal nerve blocker to reduce hunger.

# Food Addiction and the Reward Centers of Your Brain

Your brain has a pleasure center that identifies enjoyable experiences and reinforces the desire for you to repeat the same pleasurable action. This reward circuit responds to all sorts of pleasure, from laughter to sex, food to drug highs. The reward pathway evolved to promote activities that are essential to survival by driving our feelings of motivation, reward, and behavior. The same pathway is at the root of addiction as well.

The hypothalamus is at the center of the brain's food signaling process. In addition to monitoring the body's available energy supply by detecting leptin and blood sugar levels, the hypothalamus is

Alexis, at sixty-three, had watched her weight creep up in small incre-ments over the years. She had become a "professional dieter" and she repeatedly regained more than she had lost. Having weighed 120 pounds when she got married forty years ago, she now weighed 204 pounds. She decided this could not continue and came to see me. She was five feet three inches and had a BMI of 36. She told me she was hungry all the time and that she craved sugar day and night. Chocolate cake and brownies were her downfall. Even when she was full after a meal, she had to have a sweet dessert. Alexis felt she could begin to take control of her weight if she could break her addiction to sweets.

Before doing anything else, I put her on two 500mg pills of metformin a day. She came back for her next appointment in a state of elation. In just two weeks on the medication, her hunger was gone. After years of struggle, her cravings had stopped being a problem. She hoped the other changes she was going to make in her life would have such dramatic re-sults, but was convinced that she could get her weight down to a healthy level by the time she was sixty-five. She didn't want to become old before her time. We worked together to help her reach her weight goal once she jump-started her weight loss by breaking her sugar addiction.

connected to the reward pathways. It is wired to areas in the brain that control taste, reward, memory, emotion, and decision-making in a circuit that controls the drive to eat.

If you are hungry and someone puts a sandwich in front of you, your five senses send signals to your brain that there is something to eat. Stored in your brain are memories that tell you you will feel good when you eat the sandwich and that your hunger will disap-pear. Your brain instructs you to pick up the sandwich and eat it. As your senses inform the brain that your stomach is filling up with good-tasting food, your brain releases the neurotransmitter do-pamine, which gives you a jolt of pleasure, a reward for eating the sandwich. Not only do you feel good when you do something ben-eficial, but the reward pathway makes sure you repeat the behavior whenever possible by connecting regions of the brain that control memory and behavior. By creating the memory that eating makes you feel good, you are more likely to repeat the behavior that is necessary for your survival.

This reward circuitry developed in our ancient ancestors when starvation was a common cause of death, because food was scarce. In our current food-abundant environment, it is easy to be stimulated to eat, even when hunger is not an issue. The urge to eat can be suppressed by signals from the executive decision-making centers of the brain. The ability to override brain-reward signals can be impaired in people who are obese.

**Foods that are rich in sugar, fat, and salt affect your brain in the same way as alcohol, nicotine, heroin, and cocaine do.** Highly palatable foods trigger the release of endorphins and feel-good brain chemicals such as dopamine. Once people experience the pleasure associated with increased dopamine transmission in the brain's reward pathway from eating certain foods, they feel the need to eat again. The reward signals from highly palatable foods may override other signals of fullness and satisfaction. As a result, people keep eating even though they are not hungry.

A study in rats suggested that high-fat, high-calorie foods affect the brain in much the same way as cocaine and heroin. When rats consume these foods in great quantities, they develop compulsive eating habits that resemble drug addiction. Doing drugs or eating too much junk food gradually overload the brain's pleasure centers. Achieving the same level of pleasure or just feeling normal requires increasing amounts of the drugs or food. In animal experiments, rats developed a tolerance to the pleasure the food gave them, and they had to eat more to get that dopamine high.

The same thing appears to happen to people. Frequent consumption of highly processed foods seems to be addictive in many people. Once addicted, people develop a tolerance to the food. They eat more and more, only to find that food satisfies them less and less. In a sense highly processed food affects us like an addictive drug. The ingredients in refined, modern convenience food can cause people to eat unconsciously and unnecessarily. Highly processed foods have the greatest impact on your brain, possibly by overloading hypothalamic nerves as I described earlier. Combinations of sweets and fat or starch and fat appear to be the key offenders. The more refined or processed a food is, the more rapidly its calories are absorbed, the more habit-forming it can become. Similar to addictive substances, increased amounts are needed over time to satisfy cravings and avoid symptoms of withdrawal.

The biological process is identical to what happens in your appetite center. An excess of highly caloric, processed foods causes young neurons in the reward center of your brain to die prematurely, leading to fewer neurons that don't function as well to conduct the signals, which results in a loss of sensitivity to food stimulants. You start to need more and more sugar in your blood to feel good. With the increasing need for food that will break down quickly into sugar, you will eat more and more food, and your weight will steadily rise. **The Change Your Biology Diet gives you a way to withdraw from your food addictions, leaving you satisfied with foods that feed your brain with a steady supply of energy, and that will diminish and eventually do away with your food cravings.**

## The Microbiome: A New Frontier

A new focus of attention is on the microbiome, the microorganisms that inhabit the human body. Your body is home to many more bacterial than human cells—approximately 100 trillion bacterial cells. We coexist with, adapt to, and benefit from this inner ecosystem. In the past, the count indicated there were ten times more microbial cells than human cells in the body, which was based on an estimate of 10 trillion cells in the human body. According to the American Academy of Microbiology, more recent estimates suggest that the body is composed of about 37 trillion human cells. With these revised figures, the average human body has three times more bacterial cells than human cells. The microbiome also includes viruses, fungi, and other organisms. The community is very dynamic, changing under different circumstances.

There is a microbial community wherever the body is exposed to the outside world. The skin, the linings of nasal passages, lungs, and digestive and urogenital tracts each have their own microbiome. All the microbiomes are in constant communication with the immune system to protect against pathogens, organisms that can hurt us. The intestine and colon house one of the densest microbial communities ever observed, because of their convoluted surfaces, which would be the area of a tennis court if flattened out.

The human GI tract is predominantly an ecosystem of bacteria, which can be considered a hidden organ. The gut microbiome is an efficient bioreactor that helps to extract energy and nutrients from the food we eat. **The chemical reactions that are carried out by microbes help humans digest compounds they could not break down on their own.** The gut microbiome has complex effects on human metabolism and changes in its composition have been linked to diseases including inflammatory bowel disease, autoimmune disorders, diabetes, and, of particular concern, obesity.

Gut microbes are very active metabolically. They regulate energy balance not only by extracting calories for otherwise inaccessible components in our diet, but also promote storage of extracted energy in fat cells. The metabolites they secrete pass through the gut wall into the bloodstream and circulate throughout the body.

Some of the bacteria in your gut can make you obese. There are two main groups of bacteria that could influence your body weight: bacteroidetes and firmicutes. There is evidence that obesity is associated with changes in the relative abundance of these two dominant bacteria. Obese mice and humans have a less diverse milieu of gut bacteria, with a greater proportion of firmicutes to bacteroidetes in their intestines. The ratio increases in animal experiments if they are fed high-fat diets and falls if they eat low-fat diets. The obese microbiome appears to have an increased capacity to harvest energy from the food that we eat.

Studies have shown that this trait can be transmitted from one animal to another by transferring the bacteria. If germ-free mice, which have no microorganisms living in or on them, are colonized with an obese microbiota, they overeat, gain weight, and display a significantly greater increase in total body fat compared to mice colonized with lean microbiota. Mice that are maintained in a microbiome-free state are leaner than mice that have gut bacteria even when they are fed more high-fat, high-sugar food. Without a microbiome, much of the food passes through the intestines undigested. When germ-free mice are inoculated with the microbiome of an obese mouse or human donor, they gain more fat than those that receive the microbiome of a lean donor when both receive the same amount of food. A single day of eating a high-fat diet changes the composition of the microbiome in mice. When the high-fat microbiome is transferred to a germ-free mouse, that mouse will gain weight. These studies suggest that there are strong feedback loops that connect diet, the microbiome, and metabolism.

Increased intake of dietary fiber has been associated with reduced appetite and weight loss. This effect starts in the microbiome. Microbes in the gut ferment fiber in the colon and create short chain fatty acids, which stimulate the release of the gut hormones peptide YY (PYY) and glucagon like peptide-1 (GLP1). These are satiety hormones that make you feel full. In mice, propionate is the most active short chain fatty acid. When mice received a transplant from a donor with a gut microbiota that produces elevated levels of propionate in the colon, they have lost weight and reduced body fat. A recent human study shows a similar effect. When propionate is delivered directly to the colon, PYY and GLP-1 increase dramatically, which reduces the desire to eat, prevents weight gain, and reduces abdominal fat in overweight adults. The use of propionate as a dietary treatment for obesity needs to be explored. If we could stimulate the production of propionate with targeted dietary fibers, we might be able to prevent weight gain.

The microbiome has become a big area of science. The question is, can patients take a probiotic to lose weight? The answer is soon, but not just yet. **Prebiotics, fibers which encourage the growth of beneficial bacteria, can be used for stimulating the growth of a weight-losing microbiome** in the gut, but as far as giving probiotics, specific bacteria, to encourage weight loss, it takes time to find a mixture that encourages the growth of beneficial microbes, and this is a new area of study. Expect some important breakthroughs in weight management to come from research in this area.

. . .

The chapter that follows shifts focus from what is happening inside your body to what you can do to correct the damage your diet has done to your internal weight control systems. Winning the Hunger Games lays the groundwork for change that will deliver the results you have previously tried to achieve without success—dropping pounds permanently.

# PART 2

# The Change Your Biology Program

CHAPTER 4

# Winning the Hunger Games

IT PROBABLY ISN'T NEWS TO YOU that you should avoid eating too much food that is high in sugar, starch, and fat if you want to lose weight. But now you are aware of the toll your body pays for eating too much of those things: damage in the neurons of the appetite control and reward centers in your brain, disruption of communication from insulin and leptin resistance, the vagus nerve and gut microbiome, increased fat storage, and decreased metabolic rate. Those biological changes undermine your efforts to control your weight. You can break through these barriers to weight loss by committing to dietary changes that will provide your body with the steady supply of energy it needs to function well and to avoid caloric power surges and the ups and downs of the blood sugar roller coaster.

There is so much noise out there about the best diet for weight loss. As you saw in "A Brief History of Diets" (page 7), most fad diets involve drastic caloric reduction. The trends shift from low fat to low carb and back again. First, let's take a look at the differences among the most common diets.

## Talk to Your Doctor Before Starting a Diet

Before starting a diet, always talk to your doctor and review the medications and supplements you are taking. The dosage for some of your medications may need to be adjusted if your food intake changes. Dieting can affect certain conditions and medical treatments. Here is a brief overview for quick reference, so that you can discuss these issues with your health care provider:

Diabetes: If you use insulin or sulfonylureas (such as Glucotrol, or Amaryl) to treat your diabetes, you will need a reduction in medication to avoid low blood sugar. Changes should be made at the beginning of the program to prevent hypoglycemia (low blood sugar). Other diabetes medications may also require adjustment.

Congestive Heart Failure, Coronary Heart Disease, Hypertension, and Kidney Disease: Weight loss usually produces a diuretic effect. As a result, if you are taking a diuretic, the dose will probably have to be reduced. In addition, other medications will have to be tapered. Blood thinners (Coumadin) may need adjustment because of increased vegetable intake, which reduces their effectiveness.

Cancer: Having cancer should not prevent you from losing weight if you need to, especially with cancers of the breast, prostate, and colon. Intentional weight loss may not be appropriate if cancer is active. The risk versus the benefit of weight loss should be evaluated carefully.

Epilepsy (Seizure Disorder): Serum levels of medical treatments for epilepsy such as phenytoin, phenobarbital, and carbamazepine may vary with diet changes.

Gastrointestinal Disorders: Digestive tract disorders may be aggravated by the increase in dietary fiber in your diet. In most cases this is temporary. You should follow the dietary recommendations for your gastrointestinal disorder. Vitamin absorption may be affected, either increased or decreased.

**Depression and Mood Disorders:** Serum levels and the effectiveness of medications such as lithium and MAO inhibitors can be affected by diet.

Losing weight is a full-body experience. As you have seen in the previous pages, complex interactions of various mechanisms are involved. It is important to be certain that an existing condition does not complicate your efforts.

......

- **Low fat** is clear: a diet that severely limits the amount of fat consumed, especially saturated fat, cholesterol, and total caloric intake. A low-fat diet focuses on vegetables, fruits, fish, and chicken, reduced fat dairy products, with some leeway for simple carbohydrates.

- **Eating a high-protein diet can make you less hungry.** The diet focuses on protein sources that are nutrient rich and low in saturated fats, avoiding simple carbohydrates, with a focus on lean meats, fish, low-fat dairy products such as unsweetened nonfat to 2% yogurt, and legumes.

- A **low-carbohydrate** diet focuses on protein, fats, leafy vegetables and limited quantities of other vegetables, and some fruit, and totally eliminates pasta, potatoes, rice, bread, crackers, and baked goods. A low-carb diet may be more effective than low glycemic, but it is harder to comply with.

- A **low-glycemic** diet is a form of low-carbohydrate diet, but it is easier to follow, because you can eat a larger range of complex carbohydrates such as vegetables, fruit, some whole grains and multigrain starches, including whole-grain bread, pasta, and cereals. A low-glycemic diet does measure carbohydrate intake based on how long it takes a food to be digested—in other words, how much and how quickly blood sugar will increase after carbs are eaten. You will read more about how the glycemic index of a food is measured in the next chapter.

- The **Mediterranean** diet is usually identified as a heart-healthy eating plan. It is a balanced diet that focuses on eating plant-based foods such as vegetables, fruits, whole grains, legumes, and nuts, replacing butter with olive oil, using herbs and spices instead of salt, and limiting red meat.

**The truth of the matter is that when calorie intake is controlled, whether you eat a low-fat, high-protein, low-carb, low-glycemic, or Mediterranean diet does not make that much difference in weight loss.** Several studies have been conducted to compare these diets and found weight loss on the five regimens can be reasonably close. Some studies have shown that lower-carbohydrate diets have more favorable effects on cholesterol and triglyceride levels and on blood sugar control than low-fat diets do. With weight loss being equal, these findings suggest that metabolic considerations and personal preference might point to the most effective diet for you. If you are insulin resistant, especially if you have metabolic syndrome as described on page 14, a low-carbohydrate diet might be in order.

**Health issues aside, the best diet is the one you like best and find easiest to follow.** One size does not fit all when it comes to diets. When I work with a patient to customize a weight loss program, flexibility allows us to design a plan we can modify at various stages to get better results. That said, studies have shown that a high-protein/low-carb diet has the greatest metabolic effect, as you will soon learn. In this chapter, my goal is to give you some tools for taking charge of how you eat so that you can make good progress in solving your weight problems. I want to give you the information you need to make the right food choices for you, so that you find a satisfying way to eat all the time, not just while you are dieting. Later in the chapter, you will see a comparison of diets and their effects on metabolism and weight loss maintenance.

# Breaking Away from the Standard American (or Western) Diet

The standard American diet, also known as SAD, is high in animal fats, sugar, starch, salt, and a wide variety of chemical additives and preservatives, and is low in fresh fruit and vegetables. Processed food, which is 70 percent of the SAD, is loaded with fat, sugar, and salt and lacks natural fiber, vitamins, and minerals. Highly refined food has had the life processed out of it and is far removed from its original, natural state.

**Sugar is one of the most commonly used food additives in America, because it improves the taste of foods and drinks.** Added sugars are most commonly regular table sugar, called sucrose, or high-fructose corn syrup, which is found in sodas, breads, and other processed foods. The average American consumes about three pounds of sugar a week and an astronomical 130 pounds a year. To put this in perspective, at the end of the 1700s, sugar consumption was less than twenty pounds a person a year. By the end of the 1800s, sugar consumption had risen to sixty-three pounds annually. A century later, we are up to more than twice that number. We have consumed an average of 150 to 300 more calories a day during the past thirty years, 50 percent of which comes from sodas, energy drinks, sweetened iced teas, fruit juices, and other beverages, without changing our level of physical activity to compensate for the additional calories. **Added sugar is one of the dietary excesses that is driving the obesity epidemic.**

The American Heart Association recommends that women limit their sugar intake to no more than six teaspoons a day, which provides about 100 calories. Men's sugar limit is no more than nine daily teaspoons, or about 150 calories. To put these recommendations in perspective, a twelve-ounce can of soda contains 140 calories from sugar, or about ten teaspoons. That's right—your daily recommended sugar intake is less than or equal to one can of soda a day, depending on your gender. **The average adult consumes about twenty-two teaspoons a day, more than twice what is recommended.**

## *Sugar Goes by Many Names*

Food manufacturers call sugar many things and often use several different kinds of sugar to disguise how much sugar is actually in a product. By using different sugars in smaller quantities, no one sugar finds a place at the top of the ingredients list. Below you will find an extensive list of some of the names for sugar that show up on lists of ingredients. Some actually sound healthy, but don't be fooled. Sugar is sugar, whatever they call it.

- agave nectar
- barley malt
- beet sugar
- blackstrap molasses
- brown rice syrup
- brown sugar
- buttered syrup
- cane juice
- cane juice crystals
- cane sugar
- caramel
- carob syrup
- caster sugar (superfine sugar)
- coconut sugar
- corn sweetener
- corn syrup
- corn syrup solids
- crystalline fructose
- Demerara sugar
- date sugar
- dextran
- dextrose
- diastatic malt
- ethyl maltol
- evaporated cane juice
- fructose
- fruit juice
- fruit juice concentrate
- galactose
- glucose
- glucose solids
- golden sugar
- golden syrup
- grape sugar
- high-fructose corn syrup
- honey
- invert sugar
- lactose
- malt syrup
- maltodextrin
- maltose
- mannitol
- maple syrup
- molasses
- muscovado sugar
- oat syrup
- panela
- penuche
- raw sugar
- refiner's syrup
- rice bran syrup
- rice malt
- rice syrup

- saccharose
- sorbitol
- sorghum syrup
- sucrose
- sugar
- sugar alcohol

- syrup
- treacle
- tapioca syrup
- turbinado sugar
- yellow sugar
- xylose

If you see an ingredient that ends in "–ose," it's sugar. When sugar is listed as one of the first three ingredients on a food label, put it back. That product is not for you. If you can identify more than one type of sugar on the label, avoid it. You do not need that much added sugar in your diet.

In 1822, we ate the equivalent of the amount of sugar in one twelve-ounce can of soda every five days. Today, we eat that much sugar every seven hours. Our sugar consumption has gone over the top. Reducing the amount of sugar you consume is imperative. These are the foods you should stay away from:

- Soft drinks—especially supersized ones!
- Fruit juices
- Baked goods, which are high in refined carbohydrates as well as sugar
- Candy
- Canned fruits with syrup
- Dried Fruits
- Processed foods labeled "Low-Fat"—if the fat is removed, the food is usually high in sugar.

Processed food can be addictive. All the sugar, fat, and salt it contains stimulates your brain's reward centers. You need to eat more and more of it to feel satisfied. You can become a high-flavor addict because of a processed food's intense sweetness or saltiness. Sugar and salt are added to replace the flavors that have been processed out of the ingredients. When you add more whole, fresh food to your diet, you might have to adjust to the subtle flavors of food that is alive and not doctored to make you crave it.

Risking your health is a big price to pay for the convenience of eating packaged or fast food. Eating fresh food, simply prepared, is the best way to go. This is a lifestyle change you should aspire to. As you are launching your weight loss program, you have to be practical and do what will help you lose weight. I'm not going to suggest that you change everything overnight, unless you prefer to jump right into it.

# Three Simple Sugars: Sucrose, Glucose, and Fructose

Glucose, fructose, and sucrose are called simple sugars. They are found naturally in whole foods and are added to processed foods. One is not more caloric than another. Though your tongue doesn't taste the difference among these simple sugars (though fructose *is* sweeter), your body distinguishes one from the other and uses them differently. Monosaccharides, composed of only one sugar unit, are the simplest form of carbohydrates. Glucose and fructose are monosaccharides that link together to form sucrose or table sugar, a disaccharide, half fructose and half glucose. Sucrose, obtained from sugar cane or sugar beets, is also found in fruits and vegetables.

When you eat table sugar or sucrose, it is broken down to glucose and fructose. Each is taken up by a different transport mechanism. Glucose is used as an energy source that fuels the muscles and brain and stimulates insulin release. Contrary to popular belief, fructose is not used as ready energy. The insulin produced in response to the circulating glucose stores the unused energy from fructose in fat cells. Glucose is the body's preferred source of energy. Your body processes most carbohydrates you eat into glucose, which is either used immediately for energy or stored in muscle cells or the liver as glycogen for future use.

**Since fructose is not used as an energy source for the muscles and the brain, it has a different metabolic pathway.** Fructose is only metabolized in the liver. When the liver metabolizes glucose, feedback mechanisms stop the liver from absorbing too much.

Those mechanisms do not exist for fructose. When the liver metabolizes too much fructose, increased fat production, blood sugar, and insulin resistance can result. **Studies have shown that fructose produces smaller increases in appetite-suppressing hormones like leptin. This form of sugar produces more fat than glucose, particularly visceral fat.**

Found naturally in many fruits and vegetables, fructose is added to various beverages such as fruit-flavored drinks and sodas, usually in the form of high-fructose corn syrup. Almost all fruits are a mix of fructose, glucose, and sucrose, in much lower amounts than are found in processed foods. Agave nectar, which has become a popular alternative sweetener, is mostly fructose. Though fructose increases central fat, decreases insulin sensitivity, and increases cholesterol in overweight and obese people, glucose also increases fat, mostly subcutaneous, and bad cholesterol. High-fructose corn syrup found in soft drinks is considered the enemy, but here's a revelation: the high-fructose corn syrup used in sweetened drinks and many foods in the United States is composed of 55 percent fructose and 45 percent glucose. Is this enough to make it worse than sucrose? The jury is still out. Though the evidence is growing that fructose appears to be worse for you than glucose, neither is good for you if your goal is to lose weight.

## Good Carbs/Bad Carbs

The National Health and Nutrition Examination Surveys indicate that from 1974 to 2000, carbohydrates in men's diets rose from 42 to 49 percent, and 45 to 52 percent in women's diets. This increase in ready fuel consumption accompanied by the overall decrease in activity is a major contributor to diabetes, weight gain, and obesity.

The two main forms of carbohydrates—simple and complex—are distinguished by their chemical makeup and how your body uses them. Simple or "bad" carbs are simple sugars and starches that are easily digested and raise your blood sugar levels very quickly. Soda, sweets, cookies, white food such as bread, pasta,

I saw a new patient just as I was putting the finishing touches on this book. Kim is a well-known figure in the theater. Five feet eight inches tall and weighing 275 pounds, she was tired of being the heaviest woman in the room. She had run into a friend at an opening night party and noticed how trim he looked. Kim asked him what he'd been doing. It so happened that he was a patient of ours. He told her to "go see this guy," and here she was.

She was certainly aware of how to eat and did work out with a trainer when she had the time, but found it hard to establish a regular schedule because of her work demands. As I looked at her history, I immediately saw that she was taking two medications that could promote weight gain. She was forty-seven and had begun taking progesterone to smooth out peri-menopausal symptoms. She had restless leg syndrome, a disorder that disturbed her sleep, and was taking Mirapex for it. Taking both drugs could have been contributing to her weight gain. In addition to the two drugs, she consumed a lot of carbs, starting with oatmeal every morning. She started to eat more frequently, replaced the oatmeal with eggs, yogurt, and protein shakes. She started to take her own snacks to work. When eating out, which she did often, she learned to order simple meals — grilled chicken or fish with steamed or grilled vegetables.

No matter how many people we treat, helping patients find their way is always an exciting challenge.

and rice, and low fiber foods are all sweet or starchy. When you eat these foods, your blood sugar spikes, your pancreas produces a lot of insulin to handle the circulating sugar, and some of it is stored in fat. Complex or "good" carbs are usually thought of as starches combined with fiber, the more fiber the better, providing you with a steady, even stream of energy. **The fiber in complex carbs, such as brown rice, whole grains, beans, and most vegetables, can slow down the digestion and absorption of carbohydrate.** Since complex carbohydrates do not stimulate as much insulin release as simple carbohydrates, there may be less fat storage. Processing has an impact on the absorption of carbs, so that instant oatmeal is very rapidly absorbed because it is flat and has a greater surface area and is also highly processed, while steel-cut (Irish) oatmeal is round and has much less surface area, and the starch is surrounded in part by fiber and has to be cooked from scratch. Importantly, cooking complex carbs less, or al dente, so that they are not as soft, slows down the absorption of their glucose.

In the 1980s, Dr. David Jenkins, a nutrition scientist at the University of Toronto in Canada, developed the glycemic index, a way of measuring the effect of eating carbohydrates on blood sugar. He compared how quickly and how high blood sugar rose after subjects ate the carbohydrates in certain foods compared to eating pure sugar or glucose. He gave glucose a score of 100. Foods that increased blood sugar more than glucose rated scores higher than 100 on the glycemic index. Those with smaller effects were scored under 100. Potatoes, which are considered complex carbohydrates, raised blood sugar levels almost as much as glucose. The smaller the glycemic index (GI) number, the less impact the food has on blood sugar.

**If you want to win the hunger games and feel full longer, you have to eat foods with a low GI.** Aside from delivering a steady supply of energy, lower GI foods alleviate hunger and help to control appetite. When you eat foods that are low GI, you have less chance of storing extra glucose as fat, and instead tend to store more sugar in the muscles, where it is easily burned for energy. Generally speaking, when a fruit or vegetable is very sweet, the GI is higher. The higher a food's GI, the more insulin is produced, and consequently, fat storage is heightened. This is the scale for GI:

- **Very Low GI:** less than 20
- **Low GI:** 20–55
- **Medium GI:** 56–69
- **High GI:** 70 and above

## High Glycemic Foods to Avoid or Minimize

| | |
|---|---|
| Foods containing sugar | honey, molasses, corn syrup |
| Fruits | bananas, melons, pineapple, raisins |
| Vegetables | potatoes, corn, beets, turnips, parsnips |
| Breads | all white breads, all white flour products including pasta, corn breads |
| Grains | white rice, rice products, millet, corn, corn products |
| Pasta | especially thick, large pasta shapes and brown rice pasta |
| Snacks | potato chips, corn chips, popcorn, rice cakes, pretzels |
| Alcohol | beer, liqueurs, all liquor |

If you want to check the glycemic index of a food, you can go to the website www.glycemicindex.com. Eating low-glycemic food will jump-start your weight loss.

Later on, the glycemic index was modified to take into account a typical portion of the product consumed. This led to the development of the term "glycemic load." Glycemic load measures the amount of carbohydrate in a food and the impact of that carbohydrate on blood sugar levels. The glycemic load is determined by multiplying a food's glycemic index as a percentage by the amount of carbohydrates it contains. The scale of glycemic load measurements is as follows:

- **Low Glycemic Load:** 10 or under
- **Medium Glycemic Load:** 11–19
- **High Glycemic Load:** 20 or above

This is a list of representative foods to give you a sense of where foods fall on both scales. Remember, the lower a food's glycemic index or glycemic load, the less it affects blood sugar and insulin levels. Some foods, such as watermelon, have a high glycemic index, because of the carbs they contain, but a low glycemic load. The carb level is not high in a serving, because of watermelon's large water content. In other cases the glycemic index is lower, but the average portion is larger. Glycemic load supersedes glycemic index when you are evaluating a food. Here is a list of common foods to give you an idea of how this works:

| Food | Glycemic Index | Glycemic Load |
|---|---|---|
| **Breads 1 ounce serving = 1 slice** | | |
| Corn tortilla (6 inches) | 52 | 12 |
| French bread | 95 | 13 |
| Hamburger bun | 61 | 12 |
| Kaiser roll | 73 | 12 |
| Rye bread | 65 | 9 |
| New York white bagel (4 ounces) | 72 | 40 |
| White pita bread | 68 | 10 |
| Whole grain bread | 51 | 7 |
| Whole wheat bread | 71 | 9 |
| **Vegetables** | | |
| Baked white potato (medium) | 111 | 33 |
| Baked sweet potato (medium) | 70 | 22 |
| Broccoli, cabbage, celery, cauliflower, green beans, mushrooms, spinach (unlimited) | 0 | 0 |
| Carrots (1 medium) | 35 | 2 |
| Corn on the cob | 60 | 20 |
| Green peas (½ cup) | 51 | 4 |
| Parsnips (1 medium) | 52 | 4 |

| Food (continued) | Glycemic Index | Glycemic Load |
|---|---|---|
| **Fruits** | | |
| All berries (1 cup) | 40 | 5 |
| Apple (medium) | 39 | 6 |
| Banana (medium) | 51 | 12 |
| Cantaloupe (1 cup) | 65 | 4 |
| Grapefruit (half) | 25 | 3 |
| Grapes (1 cup or 25 small) | 59 | 11 |
| Orange (1 medium) | 48 | 7 |
| Peach (medium) | 28 | 2 |
| Pineapple (1 cup) | 66 | 12 |
| Raisins (1 small box) | 64 | 21 |
| Tomato (medium) | 38 | 2 |
| Watermelon (1 cup) | 72 | 5 |
| **Nuts** | | |
| Almonds, hazelnuts, macadamia nuts, pecans (limited because of fat content) | 0 | 0 |
| Cashews, salted | 27 | 3 |
| **Beans and Legumes (½ cup cooked)** | | |
| Chickpeas | 28 | 5 |
| Hummus | 6 | 0 |
| Kidney beans | 29 | 7 |
| Lentils | 29 | 4 |
| Pinto beans | 39 | 6 |
| Soy beans | 15 | 1 |
| **Grains (½ cup cooked)** | | |
| Brown rice | 55 | 10 |
| Bulgur | 48 | 12 |
| Quinoa | 53 | 7 |
| White rice | 64 | 16 |

| Pasta (½ cup cooked) | | |
|---|---|---|
| Spaghetti, white | 46 | 11 |
| Spaghetti, whole wheat | 42 | 9 |
| **Beverages (1 cup)** | | |
| Apple juice, unsweetened | 44 | 30 |
| Cola | 63 | 16 |
| Orange juice, unsweetened | 50 | 12 |
| Tomato juice | 38 | 4 |
| **Snacks** | | |
| Microwave popcorn (1 cup) | 55 | 6 |
| Pretzels (1 ounce) | 83 | 16 |

Since the range of glycemic load is small, it is most helpful to look at the glycemic index of a food in conjunction with the glycemic load.

# Fat Is Not the Enemy

For years, the dietary buzzwords have been "fat-free" and "reduced-fat" for weight loss and lowering the risk of cardiovascular disease. Years of low-fat diets have failed to produce the desired results of controlling the diabetes epidemic, improving obesity rates, lowering the risk of heart disease, or improving general health. When people began to reduce the amount of fat in their diets, they tended to consume more carbohydrates. To create low-fat foods, food manufacturers added more sugar for flavor, which was not a healthy solution. **Now there has been a reversal in thinking about fat.** Recent studies have compared higher-protein, lower-carbohydrate diets with low-fat diets and have found that the former have more favorable effects on weight loss, body composition, metabolic rate, and cardiovascular risk than low-fat diets. **A review of current research has revealed a lack of evidence for the link between fats in the diet and risk for cardio-vascular disease.** All that concern about saturated fat and its effect on high cholesterol and triglyceride levels now appears misplaced. These findings have provoked controversy, and people are reluctant to move away from medical advice they had been following for years. I wouldn't advise you to increase the amount of saturated fat in your diet, but in my opinion, the new take on dietary recommendations is persuasive about shifting the focus of concern from fat to carbohydrates for weight loss.

**Fat does not necessarily make you fat.** Its bad reputation is partly based on the fact that fat is a concentrated source of energy with twice as many calories per gram as protein or carbohydrates. Fat has nine calories per gram compared to four calories per gram for carbohydrates and protein. Fat is even more caloric than alcohol, which has seven calories a gram. Despite being calorie dense, eating the right fat in moderation is necessary for good health. You need some fat in your diet to give you a full sense of satiety, to absorb fat-soluble vitamins A, D, E, and K, and to provide essential fatty acids, which your body does not produce. Since fats make food flavorful, filling, and create a satisfying feeling in the mouth, processed and fast foods are packed with fat to keep you eating more. At the same time, foods that are high in sugar and carbohydrates are often high in fat as well, as in ice cream, pastries, and cakes, which is the double whammy that can easily create a calorie overload.

# The Gold Standard: Extra-Virgin Olive Oil

Olive oil is an important component of a Mediterranean diet. People from that region have longer life expectancies and lower risks of heart disease, high blood pressure, and stroke compared with North Americans and Northern Europeans. Greeks consume an average of twenty-four liters per person a year, Spaniards fifteen liters, and Italians thirteen liters. In contrast, the average per person annual consumption of olive oil in the United States is one liter of this healthy dietary fat.

**Olive oil, composed primarily of monounsaturated fatty acids (MUFA), has health benefits not found in saturated and trans fats.**

Made from crushing and then pressing olives, olive oil is available in a variety of grades: extra virgin, virgin, pure, and refined. Here is how they differ:

- Extra virgin is the unrefined oil that comes from the first pressing of the olives. It has the most delicate flavor and the highest level of beneficial plant nutrients from the olive.

- Virgin olive oil is from the first pressing of the olives but is more acidic, has lower phytonutrient levels, and is less delicate than extra virgin.

- Pure olive oil is a phrase that can be misleading. "Pure" typically indicates that the oil is a blend of refined and unrefined virgin olive oils.

- Refined or "light" olive oils are lower in acidity than extra-virgin or virgin olive oils, but lose some of olive oil's unique nutrient content in the refining process. Refined olive oils can be treated with heat or diluted with less expensive oils such as soybean and canola. Solvents are sometimes used when the oil is extracted.

Extra-virgin olive oil is the way to go. An extensive list of phytonutrients are found in extra-virgin olive oil. Most important are polyphenols, which have antioxidant and anti-inflammatory effects. Extra-virgin olive oil contains more than two dozen other anti-inflammatory nutrients, which are responsible for olive oil's health benefits. Consuming as little as one to two tablespoons of extra-virgin olive oil a day has been associated with significant anti-inflammatory benefits.

With the addition of olive oil to diets low in monounsaturated fat, studies have shown that participants tend to have a decrease in their total blood cholesterol and the ratio between LDL and HDL. The high level of oleic acid in olive oil has been linked to a decrease in blood pressure. Olive oil improves the function of the lining of the blood vessels and can help to prevent blood clotting that leads

Harper is an event planner with type 1 diabetes. To control her diabetes, she requires a large amount of insulin, which caused her to gain weight. She was five feet tall and weighed 147.5 pounds. Her waist was 32.5 inches and her BMI was 27.5. She had been 120 pounds the year before she came to see me. Even though she is very active, walking, running, or biking daily, she had gained more than twenty pounds in a year.

In addition to insulin, Harper was taking Wellbutrin and thyroid medication. She was eating a low-fat diet she considered healthy. For breakfast, she would have dry toast and a bowl of fruit or yogurt and fruit with granola. She was addicted to high-carb granola bars, which she would grab while running very demanding events.

She lowered her carb intake and her insulin. I kept her on Wellbutrin and prescribed metformin. She was able to manage her blood sugar with a big decrease in the insulin she takes because of her high-protein, low-carbohydrate diet. Harper now spins and always has a high-protein snack before exercise. After eight months, she is down to 115 pounds and is determined to stay there.

to heart attacks and strokes. Taking these effects into account, extra-virgin olive oil appears to reverse metabolic syndrome. In one study, the addition of extra-virgin olive oil or nuts reduced the risk of stroke beginning immediately after the study started, making it look like a direct, almost medicinal effect, and not related to weight or other factors. Animal studies have found that cardiovascular benefits from olive oil were not achieved if the lab animals consumed too many calories and too much total food. This result suggests that olive oil has to be part of an overall healthy diet to deliver health benefits.

German and Austrian scientists discovered that **olive oil could aid weight loss by making people feel fuller for longer and by staving off hunger pangs.** They tracked five hundred volunteers who, every day for three months, ate yogurt to which either olive oil, canola oil, lard, or butter had been added. Those who had olive oil ate fewer calories overall by nearly 200 calories a day, and none gained weight or body fat. Blood tests showed they had higher levels of serotonin, a neurotransmitter that affects the perception of satiety. It appears that the smell of the oil is partly responsible for the feelings of fullness. Other studies have supported the finding that when people substitute monounsaturated fatty acid–rich olive oil for saturated fat, they ate less food and either maintained their weight or lost weight. Since fat takes longer to digest than protein and carbs, it keeps you feeling fuller longer. Several other studies indicate that monounsaturated fat enhances the breakdown of stored fat. Making extra-virgin olive oil a part of your daily diet is essential if you want to change your biology to lose weight and get healthy.

# Overview of the Change Your Biology Diet

**Taking all this science into account, the diet that appears to help my patients lose weight most successfully is a low-glycemic or low-carb Mediterranean-type diet that has plenty of protein.**

One study compared maintenance of weight loss in four groups of people and a control group who ate 800 calories a day during a twenty-six week period. All patients in the study lost at least 8 percent of their body weight. One group ate a low-protein, high-glycemic index diet; another high-protein, high-glycemic index; the third low-protein, low-glycemic index; and finally high-protein, low-glycemic index. Not only did those in the high-protein, low-glycemic index group do better, but 50 percent more continued with the program compare to the other groups. I'm including the graph that follows because it gives a clear picture of the effectiveness of different ways of eating when you are trying to maintain weight loss. Week 0 is when the diet is finished and they switched to a maintenance program, having lost an average of 24 pounds. After 26 weeks, the high-protein, low-glycemic group was down 1 pound; the low-protein, high-glycemic group had regained 3.5 pounds.

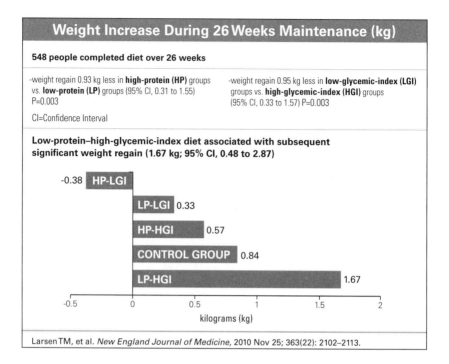

## Weight Increase During 26 Weeks Maintenance (kg)

**548 people completed diet over 26 weeks**

-weight regain 0.93 kg less in **high-protein (HP)** groups vs. **low-protein (LP)** groups (95% CI, 0.31 to 1.55) P=0.003

CI=Confidence Interval

-weight regain 0.95 kg less in **low-glycemic-index (LGI)** groups vs. **high-glycemic-index (HGI)** groups (95% CI, 0.33 to 1.57) P=0.003

**Low-protein–high-glycemic-index diet associated with subsequent significant weight regain (1.67 kg; 95% CI, 0.48 to 2.87)**

-0.38 | HP-LGI
LP-LGI | 0.33
HP-HGI | 0.57
CONTROL GROUP | 0.84
LP-HGI | 1.67

kilograms (kg)

Larsen TM, et al. *New England Journal of Medicine,* 2010 Nov 25; 363(22): 2102–2113.

You can see that eating a high protein/low glycemic index diet was best for maintenance and a low protein/high glycemic index diet had the worst results. No weight was lost. In fact, the most weight was gained in that group. The high protein/low glycemic index group lost the most weight and gained the least during the twenty-six weeks after the original weight loss. That is how you will be eating on the Change Your Biology Diet.

These are the general guidelines for the Change Your Biology Diet:

- Eat vegetables and protein before eating anything else at your meal.

- Eat more vegetables. All you can eat. Make fresh, whole food the core of your diet.

- Eat fish and poultry, or even nuts and vegetarian sources of protein as your mainstays, as they have less saturated

Since Elise, who was in her mid-fifties, had a difficult peri-menopause, she was worried about her menopausal years. Her ailing mother lived five blocks away from her, and Elise tried to visit her every day to check in with the woman who cared for her. She came for a consultation, because she was surprised to find that she was getting winded walking to her mother's place. Short of breath, she had to stop to rest along the way. She finally started to take a cab for the few blocks to her mother's apartment.

She was 5 feet 3½ inches, weighed 270 pounds, and had a BMI of 46. She had been tested for sleep apnea before seeing me, but she wasn't using her sleep machine. Her blood pressure was high, and she had fatty liver disease as well. By eating a high-protein, low-glycemic diet, and using a CPAP machine intermittently, she lost thirty-three pounds in six months. That was enough to lower her blood pressure, and she was able to go off her blood pressure medication. She was able to walk to visit her mother without getting winded.

fat. Try to limit the amount of red meat you eat to two servings a week.

- **Avoid anything white,** including bread and rolls, rice, pasta, and potatoes. When you are indulging in carbs, choose breads, pasta, crackers, and cereals made from whole grains, which still have their healthy outer coat, making them fiber-rich and slowing down their digestion.

- **If you have carbs, eat them last at your meal.**

- **Eat beans, legumes, and two servings of fruit per day to satisfy your cravings for carbs.** Eat the vegetables and protein first.

- **Have some extra-virgin olive oil every day.** It may not help you drop pounds, but it will definitely improve your health.

- **Do not add salt to your food at the table.** Enjoy the flavor of the food as it is prepared.

- **Only eat a moderate amount of dairy products,** and when you do, make sure they are low-fat. Note that I did not say no-fat. Regular milk is 3 percent fat. Two percent milk has a third less fat than whole milk. One percent milk has two-thirds less fat than whole milk. You do need some dietary fat, so I suggest you use 1 percent milk. Low fat yogurt does not have to be limited, because it appears that it reduces risk of diabetes.

- **Forget about frying food.** Bake, roast, steam, stir-fry, broil, grill, or microwave instead. If you do fry, use olive oil.

- **Use olive oil spray to coat pans or parchment paper for roasting** to reduce unnecessary fat.

- **Drink plenty of non-caloric fluids,** as much as you can, flat or carbonated, including unsweetened tea. Staying hydrated keeps your body running smoothly by maintaining the balance of your body fluids, keeps your gastrointestinal tract flowing, and may fill you up, reducing your hunger. Drinking pure water beats soda or juice any day.

This overview is an introduction to the changes you have to commit to in your diet. My patients find the prospect less daunting when they comprehend how profoundly the food they eat affects their bodies and their health. In the chapters that follow, you will find specific, day-by-day suggestions on how to eat on the Change Your Biology Diet. I want to take the guesswork out of the program by giving you all you need to know and do to start losing weight steadily.

# Portion Control in a Supersized World

If you eat out often, you can become accustomed to dinner plates heaped with food and lose all sense of proportion about what is an appropriate amount to eat. Generally speaking, eating about half of what is served to you at most restaurants is about right. You can always take the other half home. Never be embarrassed to ask the waiter to pack up your leftovers. Since it is easy to misjudge correct portions sizes, this visual reference should be a help:

| Serving | Visual |
| --- | --- |
| 1 cup | baseball |
| ¾ cup | tennis ball |
| ½ cup | computer mouse or lightbulb |
| ¼ cup | egg |
| 3 ounces chicken or meat | deck of cards |
| 3 ounces of fish | checkbook |
| 1 ounce or 2 tablespoons | golf ball or Ping-Pong ball |
| 1 tablespoon | poker chip |
| 1 teaspoon | the tip of your thumb or one die |

I will discuss in more detail in the meal plans the portion sizes that will put you on the right track to lose weight. At this point, I want you to be aware of how much you are eating. It's easy to underestimate how many calories you consume at every meal and in between, even if you are eating healthy food. In order to analyze your dietary intake accurately, you have to be able to eyeball how much you are actually eating. Without a realistic sense of whether you are overeating and by how much, you will have a hard time interpreting the results of your diet and knowing when modifying it is necessary.

• • •

This chapter has laid the groundwork for an action plan. The next chapter introduces the Breakthrough Dozen, twelve proven strategies for successful weight control. Research and our own clinical experience have identified habits that will help to reset your biological tendency to gain weight and could protect your appetite control center from damage by minimizing calorie overload.

# CHAPTER 5

# The Breakthrough Dozen: 12 Proven Strategies for Lifelong Weight Control

THE BREAKTHROUGH DOZEN ARE BEHAVIORS WE have found effective in facilitating weight loss. These strategies are an important part of the Change Your Biology plan. If you want to drop excess pounds permanently, adopting these strategies as habits, part of your daily routine as automatic as brushing your teeth, will help you to achieve your goals and win the hunger games.

1.  **Have protein for breakfast—it will reduce your appetite for the rest of the day.**

    One study served three groups of women three different breakfasts. One group had just a glass of water, while the other two groups consumed about 300 calories and equal amounts of fat and fiber. The difference was in the protein content, 3 grams for one group and between 30 and 39 grams for the other. Well into the afternoon, those who ate the high-protein breakfast reported feeling less hungry and had less desire to eat. They also ate 175 fewer calories for lunch.

    Protein is a calorie-burning, muscle-building nutrient that takes time to digest. Protein for breakfast takes longer to digest than a bagel or muffin, and that will keep you feeling full. It stimulates the secretion of peptide YY, a gut hormone that triggers feelings of satiety. Another study found that dieters who increased their protein consumption to 30 percent of their daily calories ate nearly 450 fewer calories a day less and lost about eleven pounds in twelve weeks. Starting your day with a high-protein breakfast will set you up to eat less as the day goes on.

2.   **At meals, always eat vegetables and protein first.**
     As you know, vegetables that are high in fiber and low in simple sugars are digested and absorbed slowly, which can help to control insulin response. Eating a salad or vegetables at the start of a meal will fill you up and limit the amount of protein, fat, and simple carbs you consume.

3.   **Say no to the breadbasket.** Eat carbs late in a meal and late in the day.
     The worst thing you can do is start a meal with bread. At any meal during which you plan to eat starchy food, hold off and eat it last, because you will eat less if you fill up on vegetables and protein first. But it goes beyond that. You can reduce the glycemic load of food by changing the order in which it is eaten. I am including a graph that will give you proof that you should eat your vegetables and protein first. It compares the response of eleven patients in the study.
     In this study, we gave study subjects bread at the beginning of the meal, followed by chicken and vegetables fifteen minutes later, depicted by the black line. On another day, we gave the same people the exact same meal, but this time gave the chicken and vegetables first, followed by the bread. As you can see from the graph, eating carbohydrates first causes a rise in glucose levels in the blood within thirty minutes of eating

and a spike within sixty minutes. Insulin release would accompany that spike. Eating carbs last shows a significant difference in the blood sugar levels, which rise only slightly in a two-hour period. So that's why you can "hide" your carbohydrate toward the end of your meal.

Though what I am about to say might seem counterintuitive, the later in the day you eat carbs, the easier it seems for your appetite to stay in control. I know you've heard for years that if you are going to eat bad carbs you should do so early in the day so that you burn it off. That has proven not to be true. According to researchers at Hebrew University, eating most of your carbs at night reduces daytime hunger and helped people participating in a study lose 20 percent more weight than going on a traditional low calorie diet. In the study, seventy-eight Israeli police officers were split into two groups. They went on a six-month-long

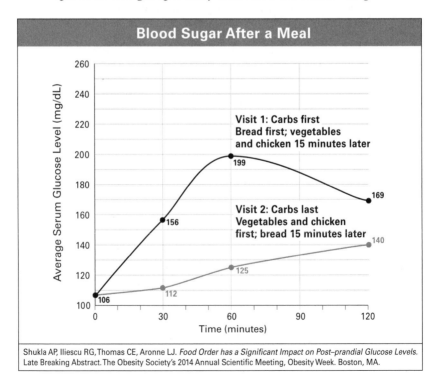

Shukla AP, Iliescu RG, Thomas CE, Aronne LJ. *Food Order has a Significant Impact on Post-prandial Glucose Levels.* Late Breaking Abstract. The Obesity Society's 2014 Annual Scientific Meeting, Obesity Week. Boston, MA.

low-calorie diet of 1,300 to 1,500 calories a day, eating equal amounts of carbs, protein, and fat during the day. Half the officers ate most of their carbs at night, while the other half ate them during the entire day. The officers who were nighttime carb eaters lost 27 percent more body fat than those in the other group. While the night carb group felt 13.7 percent fuller at the study's end, the other group said they were hungrier. The level of inflammatory hormones in the night carb group decreased by 27.8 percent compared to 5.8 percent in the dieters who ate carbs throughout the day.

Previous studies have found that concentrating carbohydrate consumption at the end of the day modifies the day-night pattern of leptin. The researchers believe that low leptin levels during daytime are remnants of evolution, when prehistoric man had to wake up and look for food. Given the abundance of food today, we no longer need that mechanism.

Waiting to eat your carbs until dinner seems to be a winning strategy.

4. **It's okay to have snacks — they can help — but avoid eating too much after dinner.**

Starving yourself and going too long without eating will only increase your appetite later in the day and make it harder to control. Why make dieting harder than it has to be? The last thing you want to do is intensify your hunger pangs. The Change Your Biology Diet is not about being hungry — it's about eating in a satisfying way that turns off your hunger switch. Though some people do well with three meals, others do best having something small in between to keep energy up and blood sugar levels even. Of course, what you eat is important. Chips, cookies, and candy will set you up for a spike and crash. You will find suggestions for delicious and satisfying snacks in the next chapter.

Many of our patients tend to snack a lot at night. A recent animal study found that time-restricted eating can prevent weight gain and protect against metabolic diseases. Restricted-time feeding refers to the window of time the subjects were allowed to eat during a twenty-four-hour period. The longer the fast, the higher the benefits were. If access to food was limited to eight or nine hours, the animals were fasting for fifteen to sixteen hours. That long a fasting period had the best results. The researchers found that time-restricted feeding not only prevented weight gain and fat accumulation, but that limiting the span of time the animals ate during the day to twelve hours or less reduced inflammation, improved glucose tolerance, reduced insulin resistance, restored healthy cholesterol levels, and improved metabolic rhythms.

Time-restricted eating has not been tested on humans yet, but the findings of the animal study do suggest that it could be another weapon in our arsenal against weight gain. Given modern life, the twelve-hour window might be hard to accomplish. If you ate breakfast at 7:30 a.m., you would have to stop eating by 7:30 p.m. You know that skipping breakfast will not work, and delaying breakfast will only make you hungrier. Until human studies have been done, it can't hurt to increase the hours you fast each night. That means no snacking after dinner and no late-night refrigerator raids, which is a good policy in any event.

5.  **Avoid eating food that comes in a box.**

Highly processed food is engineered to be addictive. Packaged, prepared food is high in sugar, fat, and salt. Sugar, in particular, creates a surge in the pleasure center of your brain, just as nicotine and cocaine do. In animal studies, sugar produces three symptoms that mirror symptoms of substance abuse and dependence: cravings, tolerance, and withdrawal.

One study has shown that given the choice, rats will choose sugar over cocaine in lab settings, because the high is more pleasurable and the reward greater. In humans, sugar has been found to be habit-forming. Not only will you crave it, but you will need to eat more and more to feel satisfied. Stay away from processed, convenience food so that you stop being a high-flavor addict.

6. **Do not drink calories.**

You already know that most people are getting much of their added sugar from beverages, including sodas, energy drinks, sweetened iced teas, and fruit juices. These are empty calories that drive your weight and BMI up. A can of soda represents all the sugar you should consume in a day.

Drink water, tea, or coffee with a little 1 or 2 percent milk instead. A glass of wine now and then is okay, but remember that alcohol is high in calories that have no nutritional value. The body can't store alcohol, so the liver metabolizes it right away. Since alcohol becomes the top priority, fats, proteins, and sugars are not metabolized as efficiently, which makes you store more calories as fat. Learn to enjoy the refreshing, clean taste of water.

7. **Only consume artificial sweeteners no more than once a day.**

Artificial sweeteners are intensely sweet — and interfere with appetite signaling. When your brain perceives you have consumed a lot of sugar and then finds the energy is not available, it sends signals that you need to eat more. Artificial sweeteners appear to increase your appetite in the end. At the same time, they have been shown to alter the bacteria in the intestine, the gut microbiome, in a way that leads to insulin resistance and contributes to glucose intolerance. How it happens, no one knows.

Patricia did very well with our program. She lost more than fifty pounds and now wants to lose a bit more. She recently told me this story about an "aha" moment she had. She and her husband had gone out for a romantic dinner to celebrate their wedding anniversary. The champagne and the tempting menu made it impossible for her not to indulge. She and her husband could not resist the warm popovers and home-baked bread, and the desserts were works of art. A bowl of berries was not going to do it for her that night. Normally, when indulging, she would savor a few bites of dessert and that would be enough to satisfy her. Her restraint flew out the window when the pastry cart was rolled up to the table. And then there were the truffles and tiny butter cookies served with the coffee. She decided to enjoy it all and not to feel guilty — a one-meal indulgence was not going to undermine her achievement.

It took her three days to get back on track. The day after her anniversary celebration, she craved sweets and carbs and found herself having to resist temptation in a way she had not for some time. She knew she had to stop the backslide. Eating a carb-heavy meal had not affected her husband at all. She came to understand that she just can't put on the brakes once she starts eating carbs. The few minutes of pleasure she had experienced were not worth the struggle that followed. She said she'd remember this particular anniversary celebration for a long time because the lesson she had learned would make a difference in her continuing efforts to stay slim.

I'm not saying that you can never have a diet soda or put a packet of sugar substitute in your coffee. For many of my patients, being able to have that calorie-free sweetness keeps them from eating a piece of cake or a candy bar. You just can't overdo it. Keep in mind that artificially sweetened soda has the equivalent of four to five packets of sugar substitute per twelve ounces. At twenty ounces, an average serving, the artificial sweetener equals eight or nine packets. Given the growing understanding of the effects that artificial sweeteners have on weight gain, it seems wise to limit how much you use so your body isn't fighting weight loss.

8. **Cook everything al dente—which means "to the tooth" in Italian.**

   Though the term is usually applied to cooking pasta, you should cook your vegetables to be firm to the bite as well. Food that's al dente takes longer to digest because the carbohydrates fiber breaks down more slowly, which extends your feeling of fullness.

9. **A little exercise goes a long way.**

   Changing the way you eat is more effective for weight loss than exercise. You have to work out hard for ninety minutes a day to lose weight, because it takes a lot of exercise to burn a modest number of calories. The more familiar you are with your routine, the fewer calories you will burn. Your body is an efficient machine and adjusts to your workout to expend less energy. As you lose weight, you need less fuel to do the same workout. But this is not a pass. You still need to exercise. For long-term weight maintenance, breaking through plateaus, and reversing fullness resistance, you have to move.

   When your scale seems stuck no matter how well you are eating, it's time to exercise. Once you start exercising and build muscle mass with strength training, you can shrink your stores of fat without a drop in leptin. Regular exercise seems to sensitize the brain to leptin, possibly by driving down triglycerides that may block leptin from reaching the appetite center.

   Muscle tissue is more metabolically active than fat. Building up your lean muscle mass will help you to maintain a healthy weight. Regular exercise reduces the weight loss–induced improvement in muscle efficiency, which will help you to break through plateaus. As you age, you have a good chance of experiencing age-related muscle loss, a condition called sarcopenia. Maintaining your lean muscle mass with resistance training will make you a healthy, calorie-burning machine.

I recommend a two-step approach to exercise—lifestyle movement and strength training. Studies have shown that simply walking distances promotes longevity. You have to build movement into your everyday life. I'm not talking about training for a marathon. Instead you have to break out of a sedentary environment and move more. Simply standing more often can make a difference. Take a walk after eating, put away the remote controls, and take the stairs instead of the elevator. I suggest ways to get moving in Chapter 10.

High-strength or resistance training is a key component of overall fitness and health. Research has shown that just a few minutes of exercising at an intensity that approaches your maximum capacity produces changes in your muscles that are comparable to those of several hours of running or bike riding. Adam Zickerman, a high-intensity workout pioneer, has created three workouts for this book geared to different levels of fitness that use this high-intensity approach. You can do these safe and efficient workouts at home in under ten minutes no more than twice a week. That's not terrible, is it? These illustrated programs can be found in Chapter 10.

Once you begin losing weight, you want to lock in that loss. Moderate movement and strength training will help you break through set points to reach your target weight and stay there. I consider exercise a medicine. If you do nothing else, become active; it is the single most effective way to improve your health.

10. **Keep a daily log of what you eat, drink, and how much you move.** You'll find it easier to stay on track if you keep a daily log on your smartphone or on paper. Dieters who keep a record of what they eat are more successful. There are several good food trackers avail-

able for free on line, including www.loseit.com and
www.myfitnesspal.com. You can find them on
our website, www.BMIQ.com. They count calories
for you.

This is the simple log we give to our patients if they
want to use paper:

## Food and Activity Diary

| Week of: | Breakfast | Snack | Lunch | Snack | Dinner | Activity |
|----------|-----------|-------|-------|-------|--------|----------|
| Monday | | | | | | |
| Tuesday | | | | | | |
| Wednesday | | | | | | |
| Thursday | | | | | | |
| Friday | | | | | | |
| Saturday | | | | | | |
| Sunday | | | | | | |

Many of my patients hate to record what they have
eaten, so we recommend they eat a low-carbohydrate
diet. If you are following a low-carbohydrate diet,
counting calories becomes less important, because
cutting carbs, sweets, and starches from your diet and
watching your portions is often enough. You can eat
a limitless amount of most vegetables and can control
your portions by familiarizing yourself with the visuals
for appropriate portion size on page 101.

**11. Weigh yourself regularly.**

Whether you weigh yourself every morning or once a week is up to you. At least 75 percent of the successful dieters on the National Weight Control Registry weigh themselves at least once a week. The registry has more than five thousand members who have lost at least thirty pounds and have kept it off for at least a year. The average weight loss for members is sixty-six pounds, which they have kept off for five and a half years.

Some of my patients find it motivating to check their weight every day. If they have lost, they are encouraged. If their weight has gone up, they are determined to be more compliant and not to cheat. If you have gained 5 percent above your lowest weight, it's time to rein in your eating and get serious again. Let's say you started at 200 pounds and lost 15 percent, or thirty pounds, and are down to 170 pounds. If you gain 5 percent of that weight—8.5 pounds—and are up to 178.5 pounds, you have to put the brakes on or you will regain all the weight you have lost. Remember that your body is resisting your lower weight. You won't want to undo all that you have achieved. Weighing yourself can make you pay attention and stay in control.

**12. If all else fails, see a doctor.**

If you follow all the lifestyle changes of the Change Your Biology Diet and still have difficulty losing weight or find yourself at a plateau you can't break through, consult with your doctor to determine if you should see an obesity medicine specialist. Obesity medicine is the newest specialty in medicine. More than one thousand physicians are now Diplomates of the American Board of Obesity Medicine and focus a significant amount of time on weight management. When we work with patients at our Comprehensive Weight Control Center at Weill Cornell, we don't give up. If one thing isn't effective, we try another approach depending on how much the patient weighs and the medical risk of his or her weight.

For many of my patients, lifestyle changes alone are not enough. Many need to take medications to support their efforts. In the past three years, four new medications have been approved by the FDA. I want to be clear that taking any of the available medications will not automatically enable you to shed pounds. You still have to eat better to lose weight, and exercise to lose and maintain the most. The medications will help you break through the physical barriers that your body has set up. For some people, especially those at medical risk, that resistance can be hard to overcome without medical assistance. If lifestyle changes plus medication are not getting you the results you want, you and your doctor might discuss bariatric surgery. Less invasive procedures have been developed, producing better and better results. The options in medications and surgery are expanding because the need for medical solutions is urgent. The final part of this book will describe medications and procedures that might be what you need to achieve lifelong weight loss.

• • •

You have a game plan for making changes in your life that will help you to lose weight. Now that you know that my recommendations are backed by hard science, you should be confident that you can change the biological factors that have been preventing you from reaching your weight goals. Most weight loss programs focus on a single diet. I give you two diets from which to choose—you have to decide which of the two you will find easier to follow.

# CHAPTER 6

# The Quick Start Change Your Biology Diet

USING MEAL REPLACEMENTS TO JUMP-START weight loss gets many of my patients on a fast track. Choosing to diet with high-protein meal replacement shakes is, at least in part, a cold turkey approach. For two meals a day at the start, you do not have to deal with food. Not having to plan, prepare, or select what you are going to eat three meals a day can be liberating. My patients tell me it is as if they are turning their backs on how they used to eat and getting a fresh start. When you substitute protein shakes for two of your three meals on the Quick Start Diet, you will be surprised to realize how food occupies your thoughts and your time. Protein shakes also provide automatic portion control. Those designed for weight loss are fortified with vitamins, minerals, and nutrients to replace what you would get in a normal meal, and the added fiber will prevent you from getting hungry. If you find that a shake is not enough, you can supplement your protein shake meals with vegetable soup, steamed vegetables, and/or a salad. You can eat those foods all day long, even when you are doing the Quick Start Diet.

Some people grab a protein bar as a meal replacement for convenience when they are on the run. In my experience, shakes are more

Brenda and her husband ran a family business in New York's Garment District. She put in long hours, skipped meals, and grabbed food when she could. She usually paid no attention to what she was putting in her mouth. At five feet two inches, she was 181 pounds, had a BMI of 30, and a thirty-nine inch waist. At forty-seven, she had developed metabolic syndrome with high blood pressure and impaired blood sugar. Her prediabetic state kept her constantly hungry. She said she had begun to snore loudly.

I prescribed metformin for her early type 2 diabetes. I also prescribed phentermine, because she was having trouble managing her hunger. The protein shakes and bars on the Quick Start Diet worked well for her. They were easy to eat on the run. From April to January, she went from 181 to 120 pounds. She lost nearly a foot from her waist circumference, which is now twenty-eight inches. A year later, she has maintained the weight loss. She is off her hypertension medication, but still has mildly impaired glucose, which we are working on. She has found a way to eat that has allowed her to break her bad habits and the medical support to make her less hungry, a winning combination for her.

satiating than bars. Make sure to drink a big glass of water when you have a bar. My patients report that they feel lighter and clearer within a few days of starting the Quick Start Change Your Biology Diet.

Meal replacement diet plans have been found to produce a higher initial weight loss than food-based plans. Studies have shown that the amount of weight you lose initially predicts your ultimate success in keeping the weight you lost off. In one study, 70 percent of those who had lost 10 percent or more of their body weight after a year maintained more than a 5 percent loss at four years. Forty percent of the participants who lost between 5 and 9.9 percent at a year maintained a 5 percent or more loss at four years. Of those who lost less than 5 percent in a year, 22 percent had maintained a 5 percent loss by year four. These numbers strongly suggest that the Quick Start Diet is worth a try, at least at the beginning of your efforts to reduce, if you want to avoid gaining back the lost weight.

You don't want to lose too much weight too fast, though. Normally, one-quarter of weight loss is muscle, three-quarters fat. If you lose weight too quickly and do not consume enough protein, half the weight you lose is fat, and half is muscle. Drinking high-protein shakes protects your muscles. Research has found that people with metabolic syndrome lost a significant amount of weight and preserved muscle mass when they followed a low-calorie, high-protein diet that included protein-dense meal replacements as compared to those who followed a conventional protein diet. The researchers concluded that a protein-enriched diet may have benefits for managing metabolic syndrome and reducing inflammation. Another study found that following a diet with one or two daily meal replacements improved weight loss and maintenance and reduced waist circumference and visceral fat.

Since it is easy to become demoralized if the pounds are slow to drop, many of my patients prefer to go this route. A quick start is a great motivator. I have outlined the Quick Start Change Your Biology Diet, a six-week, three-level diet, for quick reference. In the daily schedules, I refer to Change Your Biology meals, which include low-carb, Mediterranean-style dishes. You will find guidelines and suggestions for what to eat at mealtimes and for snacks along with two weeks of meal plans in the chapters that follow (see page 156 for the meal plans).

# The Quick Start Change Your Biology Diet

## LEVEL ONE (TWO WEEKS)
### TWO PROTEIN SHAKES A DAY

You might prefer to have your meal at lunch or at dinner. For some, going the entire day without eating a meal is difficult, while others prefer the convenience of a protein shake at lunch. And you can change it up—as long as you are prepared and plan ahead.

| Meal | Food |
|------|------|
| Breakfast | Protein shake |
| Mid-morning snack | |
| Lunch | Protein shake with soup and/or steamed green vegetables or salad with steamed green vegetables dressed with a teaspoon or two of extra-virgin olive oil |
| Afternoon snack | |
| Dinner | Change Your Biology Meal |

*Or*

| Meal | Food |
|------|------|
| Breakfast | Protein shake |
| Mid-morning snack | |
| Lunch | Change Your Biology Meal |
| Afternoon snack | |
| Dinner | Protein shake with soup with steamed green vegetables or salad with steamed green vegetables dressed with a teaspoon or two of extra-virgin olive oil |

Drink water or other noncaloric beverages, including tea, seltzer, sparkling water, or coffee, with each meal and snack. Drink as much water as you feel comfortable drinking. It's a good idea to have a glass of water when you get up and before you go to bed.

## LEVEL TWO (TWO WEEKS)
### TWO DAYS A WEEK —
### TWO PROTEIN SHAKES A DAY

| Meal | Food |
| --- | --- |
| Breakfast | Protein shake |
| Mid-morning snack | |
| Lunch | Protein shake with soup with steamed green vegetables or salad with steamed green vegetables dressed with a teaspoon or two of extra-virgin olive oil |
| Afternoon snack | |
| Dinner | Change Your Biology Meal |

*Or*

| Meal | Food |
| --- | --- |
| Breakfast | Protein shake |
| Mid-morning snack | |
| Lunch | Change Your Biology Meal |
| Afternoon snack | |
| Dinner | Protein shake with soup, salad, steamed vegetables |
| | *Don't forget to drink fluids with each meal and snack.* |

## FIVE DAYS A WEEK — ONE PROTEIN
### SHAKE AT BREAKFAST

At Level Two, you continue to have two shakes a day for two days a week. On the other five days, you replace the second shake with a Change Your Biology Meal.

| Meal | Food |
| --- | --- |
| Breakfast | Protein shake |
| Mid-morning snack | |
| Lunch | Change Your Biology Meal |
| Afternoon snack | |
| Dinner | Change Your Biology Meal |

*Make sure to drink plenty of fluids.*

## LEVEL THREE (TWO WEEKS)
### ONE PROTEIN SHAKE AT BREAKFAST

| Meal | Food |
| --- | --- |
| Breakfast | Protein shake |
| Mid-morning snack | |
| Lunch | Change Your Biology Meal |
| Afternoon snack | |
| Dinner | Change Your Biology Meal |

*Drink plenty of fluids.*

Flexibility is key. You have to customize the diet to suit you, as we would do if you were consulting with me in my office. You might want to change how long you stay at any stage. A lot depends on how much weight you are losing, the rate at which you continue to lose, and whether you find the diet too restrictive after a time. You might extend your time beyond two weeks on Level 1 because you are shedding pounds quickly and do not feel deprived. At Level 2, you might decide to alternate two-shake days with one-shake days, doing two shakes for four days and one shake for three. If you plateau at any time, go back to having two protein shakes a day. What is important is not to give up.

# The Scoop on Protein Powders

At any health food or vitamin store or grocery store aisle, you will face shelves of so many different protein powders that it might be hard to pick one. A little background will simplify the choice. There are two main categories: animal source and vegetable source protein. Animal source proteins include protein derived from milk, like whey and casein, and egg white protein. Sources of vegetable proteins include soy, rice, pea, and hemp. Animal proteins are far more popular, because they tend to taste better and are nutritionally superior.

# Animal Proteins

### WHEY PROTEIN

Whey is a complete protein derived from milk. The protein component of whole milk is 20 percent whey protein and 80 percent casein. Whey is the most popular type of protein used in protein powders, because it is one of the best tasting and the most economical. There are two varieties of whey protein:

Whey concentrate has a low lactose level and is well tolerated by most lactose-sensitive people. It has minuscule amounts of fat and carbs. Its relatively low cost makes it the bestselling type of whey protein.

Whey isolate is close to being fat-free and lactose-free. It has the highest protein concentration at 90 to 95 percent. The consistency of whey isolate tends to be thinner than whey concentrate because of the lack of fat.

Whey protein products can be made of a blend of both whey concentrate and isolate and sometimes are combined with other proteins in what are called "protein blends."

### CASEIN OR MILK PROTEIN

Casein is called milk protein because 80 percent of the protein in milk is casein. The main difference between whey and casein is that whey is absorbed quickly in the digestive system while casein is absorbed slowly and steadily. Casein helps you to feel fuller longer. On labels, casein protein is often described as calcium caseinate, the purest form of casein.

### EGG WHITE PROTEIN

Egg white protein was the most popular type of protein supplement for many years, but the milk proteins have taken over the top spot because they taste better and cost less. Egg white is very low in fat and carbs. It's a good choice for those who want to avoid dairy products.

# Vegetable Proteins

### SOY PROTEIN

Soy protein supplies all eight essential amino acids. Most vegetable proteins are not complete.

Soy is a good option for vegans, but can act as an endocrine disrupter. The isoflavones in soy have antioxidant and heart health benefits. Look for labels that read "soy protein isolate," which contains more protein, isoflavones, and less cholesterol and fat compared to soy protein concentrate. Soy has a strong flavor that is hard to mask. Preliminary findings of a small study suggest that a daily serving of soy may prevent postmenopausal women from gaining visceral fat. Studies have linked soy and breast cancer because of the phytoestrogens in soy, which can disrupt women's hormones, but the findings are inconclusive. Many of the protein bars are soy based, so if this is a concern for you, make sure you try a variety of bars.

### BROWN RICE PROTEIN

As its name suggests, this protein is extracted from rice, which, as you know, is mostly carbohydrate. What is extracted is not a complete protein and has to be mixed with other plant-based proteins. It is hypoallergenic and easily digested.

### PEA PROTEIN

Pea protein is easy to digest and has a fluffy texture. It is high in glutamic acid, which helps to convert carbs into energy and not fat. Since it is an incomplete protein, it has to be blended with other vegetable proteins.

### HEMP PROTEIN

This is a nearly complete plant-based protein. It is high in fiber and contains omega-6 essential fatty acids that fight inflammation. Some studies suggest that hemp protein may be helpful in weight loss because of its high fiber content.

I recommend whey and casein protein for my patients. In addition to their known effect in preserving muscle, they contain zinc and iron. Even if you are not vegan or don't have dairy allergies, you might want to integrate some plant-based proteins into your diet. They are easy to digest and have been shown to fight inflammation.

## What to Look for in a Protein Shake or Protein Bar

When you check out the label of protein powders, premade shakes, and bars, these are the guidelines:

200 calories or less
20 grams of protein or more
20 grams of carbs or less

Most shakes are low in fiber. You can add a teaspoon of ground flax-seeds or ground chia seeds to your protein shake to provide fiber. You may find the label "net carbohydrates" in the nutritional breakdown of some bars and shakes. Net carbohydrates refers to the total carbs minus the fiber.

Try using different meal replacements, because variety is a good thing. It is important to find a product that tastes good to you. Shakes are more filling to some than bars. Even when a shake and a bar have similar compositions, a bar tends not to be as filling. We're not certain why this appears to be so.

Some of the new bars use a fiber known as soluble corn fiber. This fiber is slightly sweet, and so it is actually a slowly digested carbohydrate. It's listed as a fiber, but adds sweetness to a product. Soluble corn fiber is what makes Quest bars so low in carbohydrate and high in fiber.

My favorite shakes are the Re Muscle Health shakes which you can order online. They have an active ingredient, fortetropin, which is derived from raw eggs. Studies have shown that the product increases muscle and reduces fat compared to a program of exercise alone. Re Muscle Health bars are the only shakes and bars with an active, muscle enhancing, ingredient.

## Recommended Protein Shakes

Please note that the nutrients may vary slightly by flavor.

| Product | Formula | Calories | Protein | Carbs |
|---|---|---|---|---|
| Atkins Advantage | Premade | 150 | 15 | 2 |
| Carnation Instant Breakfast (no sugar added) | Premade/ Powder | 150 | 13 | 16 |
| Designer Whey/ Aria | Powder | 80–100 | 14–18 | 3 |
| GNC Total Lean | Premade/ Powder | 170 | 25 | 6 |
| Glucerna Hunger Smart | Premade | 180 | 15 | 16 |
| Muscle Milk Light | Premade/ Powder | 100 | 15 | 4 |
| Myoplex Carb Control | Premade | 150 | 25 | 5 |
| Optifast (Kosher)* | Premade/ Powder | 160 | 14 | 20 |
| ProtiDiet VLC | Powder | 160 | 35 | 21 |
| Pure Protein* | Premade | 170 | 23–35 | 3 |
| Re Muscle Health | Powder | 160 | 20 | 6 |
| Unjury | Powder | 100 | 20 | 4 |
| Vega 1 | Powder | 135 | 15 | 12 |

## Recommended Protein Bars

| Product | Calories | Protein | Carbs |
|---|---|---|---|
| Atkins Advantage | 210 | 14 | 17 |
| NuGo Slim-Kosher (Gluten Free) | 190 | 16 | 19 |
| Optifast-Kosher | 170 | 17 | 19 |
| ProtiDiet/ ProtiBar | 140 | 16 | 18 |
| Quest | 190 | 21 | 21 |
| Re Muscle Health** | 250 | 20 | 23 |
| Simply Bar (Vegan, Kosher, Gluten Free) | 160 | 16 | 14 |
| Think Thin (Gluten Free) | 190 | 20 | 16 |

*Only available at a doctor's office.

**Since the bar is 250 calories, we suggest having ½ twice daily.

# Turn Your Protein Shakes into Treats

A meal replacement shake can be a simple thing, or you can turn it into a major treat without too much effort. You might be perfectly happy just mixing a scoop, which is 2 tablespoons, of protein powder with water and gulping it down. If that is the case, enjoy the convenience. If you are using a vegetable or egg white protein powder, you may want to add 1 percent milk or unsweetened almond or soy milk instead of water for a richer shake. To compensate for not chewing two meals each day, some people doctor their shakes and come up with delicious and satisfying concoctions. Of course, you have to restrain yourself and keep calories in mind. Stay away from bananas and peanut butter because they are high in calories, but there are limitless possibilities you can whip together in a blender. I'm including some of my patients' favorites to inspire you. If you do add fruit to your protein shake, that is one of the two portions of fruit you are allowed a day. These recipes will work with either fresh or frozen fruit. Using frozen fruit can save time in the morning. If you opt to use milk, remember that the number of calories in your shake will go up, but the shake will taste better. Adding ice cubes is a good way to thicken a shake.

## Mocha Pick Me Up

1 scoop chocolate protein powder
½ cup cold water
1 teaspoon granulated instant coffee
5 ice cubes

Put the first three ingredients in a blender and blend to combine. Add the ice cubes gradually and blend to thicken the shake to the desired consistency.

## A Fine Use for Leftover Coffee

1 scoop chocolate protein powder
1 cup cold coffee
3 ice cubes

Combine all the ingredients in a blender and blend together.

## Mocha Mint

1 scoop chocolate protein powder
1 cup water, 1% milk, or unsweetened soy or almond milk
1½ tablespoons granulated instant coffee
3 drops mint extract
5 to 6 ice cubes

Put the first four ingredients in a blender and blend to combine. Add the ice cubes gradually and blend until the shake reaches the desired consistency.

## Peaches and Cream

1 scoop vanilla protein powder
1 cup water, 1 or 2% milk, or unsweetened soy
   or almond milk
¼ cup frozen or sliced fresh peaches
½ teaspoon ground cinnamon
½ teaspoon ground nutmeg

Combine all the ingredients in a blender and blend together.

## Sinfully Chocolate

1 scoop chocolate protein powder
1 cup water, 1 or 2% milk, or unsweetened soy
   or almond milk
2½ tablespoons unsweetened cacao powder
2 ice cubes

Put the ingredients in a blender and blend them together.

*Note:* Unsweetened cacao powder has only 12 calories per tablespoon.

## Strawberries Dipped in Chocolate

1 scoop chocolate protein powder
1½ cups hulled strawberries
1 cup water, 1% milk, or unsweetened soy or almond milk
2 tablespoons unsweetened cacao powder
Water and/or ice

Put the first four ingredients in a blender and blend to combine. Add water and/or ice gradually and blend until the shake reaches the desired consistency.

## Black and Blue

1 scoop vanilla protein powder
1 cup blackberries
½ cup water
½ cup 0 to 2% Greek yogurt
½ cup blueberries
Water and/or ice

Put the first five ingredients in a blender and blend to combine. Add water and/or ice gradually and blend until the shake reaches the desired consistency.

## An Apple a Day . . .

1 scoop vanilla protein powder
1 medium apple, peeled and cored
1 cup water, 1% milk, or unsweetened soy or almond milk
1 teaspoon vanilla extract
½ teaspoon ground cinnamon
Water and/or ice

Put the first five ingredients in a blender and blend to combine. Add water and/or ice gradually and blend until the shake reaches the desired consistency.

## Refreshing Melon Shake

1 scoop vanilla protein powder
¾ cup frozen or fresh cubed seedless watermelon
¾ cup fresh or frozen cubed cantaloupe

½ cup 1% Greek yogurt
2 tablespoons lime juice
½ cup water
½ cup ice cubes

Put the first five ingredients in a blender and blend to combine. Add the water and ice cubes gradually and blend until the shake reaches the desired consistency

## Thick Raspberry Chocolate Shake

1 scoop chocolate protein powder
¾ to 1 cup water, 1 or 2% milk, or unsweetened soy
    or almond milk
12 raspberries
6 ice cubes

Put the first three ingredients in a blender and blend to combine. Add the ice cubes gradually and blend until the shake reaches the desired consistency.

## Berry Medley

1 scoop vanilla protein powder
5 hulled strawberries
15 blueberries
10 raspberries
1 cup water, 1 to 2% milk, or unsweetened soy
    or almond milk
4 ice cubes

Put all the ingredients in a blender and blend to combine. Add water if you want a thinner shake.

## Cherries in the Snow

1 scoop vanilla protein powder
1 cup water
10 fresh or frozen pitted cherries
1 teaspoon cherry-flavored extract
3 ice cubes

Put all the ingredients in a blender and blend to combine.

## Chocolate-Covered Cherries

1 scoop chocolate protein powder
1 cup water, 1% milk, or unsweetened soy or almond milk
10 fresh or frozen pitted cherries
1 teaspoon cherry-flavored extract
3 ice cubes

Put all the ingredients in a blender and blend to combine.

## Kiwi and Blueberry Shake

1 scoop vanilla protein
½ cup 1% Greek yogurt
½ cup blueberries
2 kiwis, quartered (no need to peel)
1 cup water

Put the first four ingredients in a blender and blend to combine. Add water gradually and blend until the shake reaches the desired consistency.

## Cinnamon Roll

1 scoop vanilla protein powder
1 cup water
1 tablespoon sugar-free instant vanilla pudding mix
¼ teaspoon ground cinnamon

¼ teaspoon vanilla extract
1 packet artificial sweetener, stevia preferred
2 drops butter-flavor extract
3 ice cubes

Put all the ingredients except the ice cubes in a blender and blend to combine. Add the ice cubes gradually and blend until the shake reaches the desired consistency.

## Coconut Almond Treat

1 scoop vanilla protein powder
1 cup water, 1% milk, or unsweetened soy or almond milk
2 tablespoons raw almonds (10 to 12 medium almonds)
1 tablespoon unsweetened cocoa powder
½ teaspoon coconut extract
4 ice cubes

Put the first five ingredients in a blender and blend to combine. Add the ice cubes gradually and blend until the shake reaches the desired consistency.

## Peachy Keen

1 scoop vanilla protein powder
1 cup water, 1% milk, or unsweetened soy or almond milk
½ peeled ripe peach, or ½ cup frozen peach
6 frozen strawberries
3 ice cubes (optional)

Put all ingredients in a blender and blend to combine.

## Old-Fashioned Lemon Square Shake

1 scoop vanilla protein powder
1 cup water

1 tablespoon sugar-free instant lemon pudding mix
½ teaspoon lemon extract (optional)
3 ice cubes

Put all ingredients in a blender and blend to combine.

## Pina Colada

1 scoop vanilla protein powder
1 cup water, 1% milk, or unsweetened soy or almond milk
¼ cup fresh or frozen pineapple chunks
1 tablespoon coconut extract
3 ice cubes

Put all the ingredients in a blender and blend to combine.

## Red Velvet

1 scoop chocolate protein powder
1 cup water
1 small beet, peeled and boiled until tender

Put all the ingredients in a blender and blend to combine.

## Harvest Pumpkin Pie

1 scoop vanilla protein powder
1 cup water, 1% milk, or unsweetened soy or almond milk
½ cup canned unsweetened pumpkin
1 tablespoon sugar-free instant vanilla pudding mix
½ teaspoon pumpkin spice

Put all the ingredients in a blender and blend to combine.

As you can see from these twenty-one recipes, with a little ingenuity you can create terrific shakes that will satisfy any cravings for sweets you might have. Have fun with this—your shakes do not have to be bland, unless you prefer them that way.

If meal replacements are not for you, the next chapter presents another diet you can try, with three full Change Your Biology meals and two snacks a day. Two weeks of meal plans are included from which you can choose your single meal a day if you decide to do the Quick Start Change Your Biology Diet. The option is yours.

# Getting Started

Whether you choose to begin with meal replacements or three low-carb, high-protein meals a day, you have to prepare for the permanent changes you are going to be making in your diet. Go through your kitchen cabinets and refrigerator and get rid of the foods that you are not going to be eating. Clear the decks. You don't need to surround yourself with temptations. Give what you can to food banks. There are a lot of hungry people in the world who would benefit from having any food at all. If you have a family and a total clean-up is not possible, make a space for yourself for the food you are going to be eating. Consider the other shelves a danger zone. In time, your partner and your family may convert to your way of eating when they see how great you look and feel.

# The Change Your Biology Pantry

Stock your shelves and refrigerator with staples for your new eating plan, including:

- Bottled mineral water

- Club soda (plain or flavored)

- A selection of teas

- Extra-virgin olive oil

- Canola oil

- Olive oil spray

- Dried or canned beans: chickpeas (garbanzos), cannellini or white beans, black beans, pinto beans, kidney beans, lentils

- Canned tuna and salmon

- Chicken, fish, seafood, and lean meats

- Nuts and seeds: almonds, walnuts, peanuts, pine nuts, cashews, sunflower seeds, pumpkin seeds

- Dried herbs and spices: coriander, cumin, oregano, curry powder, assorted chili powders, rosemary, red pepper flakes

- Eggs or egg substitutes

- Low-fat milk or unsweetened almond milk

- 0 to 2% unsweetened Greek yogurt

- Low-fat cottage cheese

- Low-fat ricotta cheese

- Low-fat cheeses, such as cheddar, mozzarella, Monterey Jack, string cheese

- Protein powder

- Protein bars

- Almond, cashew, or peanut butter

- Stevia

- Extracts: vanilla, almond, peppermint, or whatever else appeals

- A four-day supply of fresh vegetables and fruit selected from the lists on pages 138–140.

Now you are ready to nourish your body with satisfying and delicious food that will put you on the path to weight loss.

# CHAPTER 7

# The Change Your Biology Diet

IF YOU FIND THE PROSPECT of having meal replacements unappealing, have tried the Quick Start diet and could not handle it, or have followed the diet for two, four, six, or more weeks and are ready for a change, the Change Your Biology Diet is another option. This diet combines a typical Mediterranean diet with a low-glycemic, low-carb eating plan. Staying away from high-glycemic foods, which contain lots of sugar and starch, will provide your body with slow-release energy. Not only will you consume fewer calories, but your blood glucose level will not skyrocket, stimulating insulin production, storage of the excess energy in fat cells, and eventually insulin resistance. You will find that your meals hold you over longer without food cravings and hunger pangs. Eating in this way without caloric surges will give your brain time to repair damaged neurons in your appetite center, gradually decrease your dependence on sweets and treats, and allow your body to become more receptive to insulin and leptin.

I have observed there is a limit to how long my patients can go without eating simple carbs. It is not realistic to expect to be able to eliminate carbohydrates from your diet forever. Assuming you are like the thousands of patients I have treated, you will start craving starchy or sweet carbohydrates at some point. Most people lose control if they go too long without "comfort" food. The Change Your Biology Diet has a unique solution. Carbohydrates have been incorporated into the second stage of the eating plan. As you have read in the Breakthrough Dozen (page 102), it is a matter of *when* you eat your carbs. If you hold off eating the carbs on your plate until toward the end of your dinner at the end of the day, you can consume enough carbs to satisfy your cravings, but you are much less likely to overeat or binge on them as you might if you had them early in the meal or early in the day.

The Change Your Biology Diet has two stages: the first, for weight loss, followed by a plan to follow once you have approached your target weight. **Generally speaking, you should stay at Stage 1 until you have lost 10 percent of your body weight.**

## STAGE ONE: WEIGHT CONTROL

Eating for weight loss has never been so easy. When you follow the plan's simple guidelines, you will have a wide variety of delicious foods from which to choose. You will find two weeks of daily meal plans, including snacks, to show you that losing weight is not about deprivation. As your cravings for less-than-healthy foods diminish and the pounds start evaporating, you, like my patients, can experience renewed energy and optimism. Knowing that you are getting a grip on your weight problems is a great incentive for staying on plan.

When you move on to Stage 2 depends on how much weight you want to lose. You should do Stage 1 for at least two weeks, but you can wait three months before you reintroduce carbs into your diet. You should consider the shift when you have achieved a 10 percent weight loss. You can do an intermediary stage if you would like. You do not have to have two servings of carbohydrates every day in Stage 2. Some people ease their way into adding carbs to their diet and have carbs just one or two days a week to start. I guess that's Stage 1½. There is no reason to eat starchy carbs if you don't really want them. Remember, you are getting your carbs from vegetables and two servings of fruit. You will lose more weight initially without them.

Betsy had three children, ages fifteen months, four years, and six years. It's no wonder she wasn't focusing on what she was eating. She had never had to think about her weight in the past. But being a working mother with a stressful life in Manhattan and three young children had taken its toll. Her weight started to creep up slowly when she turned thirty-eight. At 5 feet 6 inches, she weighed 195 pounds and her waist circumference was forty inches. She had not lost her belly fat after her last child was born. She wasn't a terrible eater, but she did snack on cake and cookies and found herself nibbling on her kids' leftovers. She told us that she was tired of people asking her, "When are you due?" As her weight approached the two-hundred-pound mark, she reached her limit. She had to do something about it.

She spent time with the nutritionists at the center and learned the principles of the Quick Start and Change Your Biology Diets. Once Betsy knew what she had to do, she followed the diet scrupulously. For her, the weight gain was not about hunger. She was able do what she had put her mind to. She hired a trainer and worked out every day. She went from 195 to 128 pounds in one year, losing 34 percent of her body weight. She had so much loose skin that she had a skin-tightening procedure done.

When she took on more responsibility at work, she started to exercise less often and gained weight. She had continued to have high-protein breakfast shakes 80 percent of the time. She was not willing to gain her weight back and wanted to stop trending upward. She came back for help. I put her on metformin, which is used to treat diabetes but has been found to help nondiabetics to lose weight. It didn't do anything for her. She concentrated on what she ate and built more physical activity into her life. Betsy now weighs between 135 and 140 pounds, which she has maintained for five years.

## STAGE TWO: LOCK IN WEIGHT LOSS

The Change Your Biology Diet is not about being on a very restricted diet and then off it. This is a way to eat for the rest of your life. If you have dieted successfully in the past only to gain the weight back, you know how easy it is to revert to the way you used to eat. Even the most careful post-diet transition to "normal" eating can lead to excesses and backsliding. That is why you will be reintroducing well-timed, simple carbohydrates to your diet at this stage. Knowing that you do not have to eliminate that food group entirely can make it easier to sustain weight loss and your commitment to your new way of eating. At this stage, you can have two servings of carbohydrates a day after you have eaten veggies and protein, preferably with dinner.

# The Way to Eat

To help you get into the swing of things, we will lay out various foods in groups and further divide them into categories: go-to foods, those that you should eat only occasionally (say, once or twice a week), and those that you should avoid altogether.

## VEGETABLES

Vegetables are an all-you-can-eat food if they are steamed, baked, roasted or grilled with a minimal amount of oil, or raw.

| Vegetables | | | |
| --- | --- | --- | --- |
| Go-To | Artichokes | Celery | Parsnips |
| | Arugula | Cucumbers | Peas |
| | Asparagus | Dried beans | Peppers |
| | Avocados | Eggplant | Radishes |
| | Bok choy | Endive | Radicchio |
| | Broccoli | Fennel | Scallions |
| | Broccoli rabe | Green beans | Shallots |
| | Brussels sprouts | Kale | Spinach |
| | Cabbage | Lentils | Squash |
| | Carrots | Lettuces— all varieties | Swiss chard |
| | Collard greens | | Tomatoes |
| | Cauliflower | Mushrooms | Zucchini |
| | | Onions | |

| Occasional | Boiled or baked sweet potato — ½ |
| | Corn |
| | Beets |
| Avoid | Turnips |
| | White potatoes |

## MEAT AND OTHER SOURCES OF PROTEIN

Limit red meat to 1 to 2 times a week.

| Meat and Other Sources of Protein | | | |
|---|---|---|---|
| Go-To | Beans, lentils, and nuts | Fish | Shellfish |
| | Canadian bacon | Lamb | Tempeh |
| | Chicken | Lean ham | Tofu |
| | Eggs or egg whites | Seitan | Turkey |
| Occasional | Almond butter | | |
| | Canned tuna in water (high levels of mercury) | | |
| | Peanut butter (chunky version preferred) | | |
| | USDA Select or Choice grades of beef (London broil, filet mignon, flank steak, 90% lean ground beef) | | |
| Avoid | Cold cuts processed with sugar (bologna and liverwurst) | | |
| | Meats with visible fat such as pastrami | | |
| | Sugar-cured ham, bacon, or other cured meats such as hot dogs, salami, prosciutto, chorizo, and coppa | | |

## FRUITS

Limit your fruits to two servings a day.

Choose fresh fruit or frozen fruit without sugar.

| Fruits | | | |
| --- | --- | --- | --- |
| Go-To | Apples | Grapefruit | Pears |
| | Apricots | Honeydew | Pineapples |
| | Blackberries | Kiwis | Plums |
| | Blueberries | Mangos | Raspberries |
| | Cantaloupe | Oranges | Strawberries |
| | Cherries | Peaches | Watermelon |
| Occasional | Bananas | | |
| | Dried apricots | | |
| | Dried figs | | |
| | Grapes | | |
| | Papaya | | |
| Avoid | Dates | | |
| | Fruit juices (even unsweetened) | | |
| | Raisins | | |

## DAIRY PRODUCTS

Always try to eat reduced-fat dairy products. Portion sizes are:

1 cup milk or unsweetened almond or soy milk
6 ounces yogurt
1 ounce reduced-fat cheese
½ cup low-fat cottage cheese or ricotta

| Dairy Products | |
|---|---|
| Go-To | 1% cottage cheese |
| | 1% milk |
| | Reduced-fat cheese |
| | Unsweetened almond milk |
| | Unsweetened soy milk |
| | Yogurt with no sugar added |
| Occasional | 2% milk |
| | Low-fat ice cream (½ cup serving) |
| | Whole milk |
| Avoid | Chocolate milk |
| | Frozen yogurt |
| | Half-and-half |
| | Heavy cream |
| | Regular ice cream |
| | Soft serve ice cream |
| | Sweetened almond milk |
| | Sweetened soy milk |

## FATS AND CONDIMENTS

The serving sizes are as follows:

1 tablespoon oil

1 teaspoon reduced-fat cream cheese

1 tablespoon reduced-fat mayonnaise/vegannaise

1 tablespoon ketchup

1 tablespoon butter substitute

| Fats and Condiments | | | |
|---|---|---|---|
| Go-To | Extra-virgin olive oil | Reduced-fat mayonnaise | Low-sodium soy sauce (no limit) |
| | Canola oil | Reduced-fat vegannaise | Mustard (no limit) |
| | Spray oils, for coating pans | Reduced-fat cream cheese | Salsa (no limit) |
| | Infused oils, such as black or white truffle oil | Red, white, balsamic, champagne, rice, and infused vinegars such as fig (no limit) | Tabasco sauce and other hot sauces, including Sriracha sauce |
| | Sesame oil, for flavor | | Spreadable fruit with no sugar added (1 tablespoon) |
| | Trans fat–free butter substitutes | | |
| Occasional | Bottled salad dressing (2 tablespoons) | Ketchup | |
| | Butter (1 tablespoon) | Pickles | |
| Avoid | Honey | Molasses | |
| | Jam | Sugars (brown, granulated, confectioners') | |
| | Jelly | | |
| | Maple syrup | | |

## BREADS AND GRAINS FOR STAGE TWO

During Stage 1, you should avoid eating food from this category completely. When you can add simple carbs to your diet in Stage 2, you still have to be careful about what carbs you choose to eat. The serving sizes are as follows:

1 slice whole-grain bread
1 (6-inch) whole-grain tortilla
½ whole wheat hot dog or hamburger roll
⅓ cup pasta, rice, or other grains

Just remember to eat vegetables first. If you want to fill your tortilla or roll with meat, have a salad first.

My patients are sometimes confused about food labeled "whole wheat," "whole-grain," and "multigrain." The difference is in the word "whole." *Whole wheat* means that the wheat in the product is made from the entire, unrefined wheat kernel. *Whole grain* refers to any whole-grain kernel such as wheat, spelt, oats, barley, or flax. Watch out for "100% wheat," which refers to refined wheat flour in which the bran and the germ have been removed during the refining process. Most of the vitamins and fiber are contained in the bran and the germ, as well as iron, zinc, and copper. Though *multigrain* products sound healthy, the term simply means that more than one type of grain has been used. The flour can be processed, bleached, or refined in a way that removes any real nutritional value. If you do not see the word "whole" on the package, the product may not be made from the entire kernel. If you are not certain, check the ingredients list to see if the first ingredient is "whole wheat flour" or another kind of whole grain. Check the nutritional information panel and make sure you are getting 3 grams or more of fiber per serving.

Research from the UK could lead to a way to support weight control and reduce diabetes. Researchers found that when pasta is cooled after cooking, its structure changes, becomeing a "resistant starch," which, acts as a dietary fiber, and is beneficial to gut bacteria. Cooking, cooling, and reheating the pasta had a  more dramatic effect: this method reduced the rise in blood sugar by 50 percent. They are now studying other foods for the same effect.

Nicole, fifty-six, had metabolic syndrome. She was five feet eight inches and weighed 275 pounds. She had intense cravings for carbs and tended to eat a lot of them. Nicole and her husband enjoyed smoking marijuana every evening, which might have contributed to her cravings for junk food.

Since she had a high insulin level, she was already taking metformin once a day. I increased the metformin to twice a day. Initially, her cravings went away. She lost twelve pounds in a month.

When her evening cravings returned three months later, we added To-pamax to her medication. At five months, she wondered if she could stick with the diet. Nicole still smoked marijuana every night and still craved carbs. She had lost a total of thirty-seven pounds. We took her to Stage 2 of the Change Your Biology Diet, on which she could have two servings of carbs at the end of dinner. That suited her well, because her cravings were the strongest then.

She hadn't been exercising regularly and decided it was time to do a cardio-strengthening routine. After five months, she had lost a total of fifty-six pounds and 20.3 percent of her body weight, and is still losing weight.

## Breads and Grains

| Go-To | Barley | Light whole-grain breads | Whole-grain breads |
|---|---|---|---|
| | Bulgur | | |
| | Farro | Low-carb, low-fat wraps | Whole-grain brown rice (not instant) |
| | Flaxseed, oat bran, and whole wheat pitas | Quinoa | |
| | | Rye bread | Whole-grain pastas |
| | | Stone-ground whole wheat pitas | |
| Occasional | Regular pasta | | Whole wheat tortillas |
| Avoid Always | Bagels | | White bread |
| | Cookies or other baked goods | | White or instant rice of any sort |
| | Crackers | | |

### *Healthy Bread Options*

Some of my patients miss bread more than anything else when they are in Stage 1 of the Change Your Biology Diet. Remember to save your carbs until the end of a meal, preferably at dinner. While you are trying to lose weight, it is best to avoid bread for breakfast. If you really want a sandwich, make sure you eat a salad or steamed vegetables first. We've compiled a list of the best, easily accessible bread choices for you:

Arnold Whole-Grain Double-Fiber Whole Wheat Bread (1 slice)

Cedar's Whole Wheat Wraps (1 wrap)

Damascus Bakeries Whole Wheat Roll Up (1 roll up)

Fiber One 100% Whole Wheat English Muffin (1 muffin)

Joseph's Oat Bran & Whole Wheat Pita (1 pita)

La Tortilla Smart and Delicious High Fiber Tortilla (1 tortilla)

Revolution Low-Carb Bread (1 slice)

Sara Lee Delightful Wheat Bread (1 slice)

Thomas' 100% Whole Wheat English Muffin (1 muffin)

Thomas' Light Multigrain English Muffins (1 muffin)

Trader Joe's High Fiber Tortilla (1 tortilla)

Tumaro's Low-in-Carb Salsa Tortillas (1 tortilla)

# Meal-by-Meal Guidelines for the Change Your Biology Diet

This eating plan was designed to reduce hunger and promote feelings of fullness as you lose weight. As you now know, eating high-fiber vegetables followed by protein at meals has been shown to increase fullness, reduce the amount you eat, and improve blood sugar control. When you are at Stage 2, carbohydrates should be eaten in moderation at the end of a meal, preferably dinner.

### BREAKFAST

Start your day right with a protein-rich breakfast. Whatever you do, don't skip the meal that breaks your overnight fast. Doing so can lead to overeating later in the day. Sweets and starches—juice, muffins, toast, Danishes, bagels, sweetened breakfast cereals—are not on the menu. Treat breakfast like the important meal it is.

Choose one high-protein option from the following list:

| Breakfast | | | |
|---|---|---|---|
| Protein | Such as ... | Flavor with | Add one |
| Protein shake/bar | *See page 124 for recommended products and pages 126–132 for some delicious recipes for shakes.* | | |
| Dairy | 6 to 8 ounces of: 0 to 2% plain Greek or unsweetened yogurt<br>Low-fat cottage cheese<br>Low-fat ricotta | Vanilla extract, stevia, cinnamon, or unsweetened cocoa powder | 1 cup berries<br>1 cup melon cubes<br>1 medium peach sliced, or 1 medium apple sliced<br>10 almonds or walnut halves<br>2 teaspoons chunky peanut/ almond butter |
| Eggs | 1 egg plus 2 egg whites<br>½ to 1 cup egg substitute<br>4 to 6 egg whites prepared scrambled, hard-boiled, poached, or in an omelet or a frittata<br>1 cup egg white salad made with low-fat mayo | Unlimited vegetables | 1 ounce lean ham<br>1 ounce reduced-fat cheese<br>2 slices turkey bacon<br>1 turkey, chicken, or veggie sausage link |
| Cheese | 2 Babybel cheese rounds<br>2 Laughing Cow cheese wedges (light or regular)<br>2 ounces low-fat cheese | | 1 sliced small apple<br>1 sliced small pear<br>1 cup berries |

## LUNCH

If you prefer to have a lighter meal in the evening, feel free to have your main meal at midday.

| Lunch Salad | | |
| --- | --- | --- |
| **Vegetable** | **Protein — 5 ounce serving** | **Dress with** |
| Unlimited vegetables of all colors. | Skinless chicken breast | 1 to 2 tablespoons extra-virgin olive oil and vinegar or lemon juice (see salad dressings beginning on page 169). |
| | Skinless turkey breast | |
| | Fish/seafood | |
| | Tuna/chicken salad made with 1 tablespoon low-fat mayo | |
| | Turkey/chicken/soy/ veggie/fish burger without roll | |
| | Lean deli meats: turkey, chicken, or ham | |
| | Vegetarian choices: tofu, seitan, or tempeh | |
| | ½ cup legumes: chickpeas, black beans, or lentils | |
| | *Use cooking spray and/or olive oil in a mister for cooking.* | |

## DINNER

Remember to fill up on vegetables. If you are in Stage 2, eat the starchy side dishes last.

| Dinner | |
| --- | --- |
| **Appetizer:** *You can have all three if you would like.* | Soup: 1 cup clear broth or vegetable, tomato, miso, or lentil soup |
| | Salad: unlimited, with 1 to 2 tablespoons of a simple vinaigrette dressing |
| | Shrimp/seafood cocktail, with 2 tablespoons cocktail sauce |

## Dinner (*continued*)

| Vegetable: *All you can eat, steamed, baked, grilled, roasted, and raw, including:* | | | |
|---|---|---|---|
| | Artichokes | Celery | Parsnips |
| | Arugula | Cucumbers | Peas |
| | Asparagus | Dried beans | Peppers |
| | Avocados | Eggplant | Radishes |
| | Bok choy | Endive | Radicchio |
| | Broccoli | Fennel | Scallions |
| | Broccoli rabe | Green beans | Shallots |
| | Brussels sprouts | Kale | Spinach |
| | Cabbage | Lentils | Squash |
| | Carrots | Lettuces— all varieties | Swiss chard |
| | Collard greens | Mushrooms | Tomatoes |
| | Cauliflower | Onions | Zucchini |

**Protein:** *5- to 6-ounce serving, baked, steamed, broiled, grilled, roasted, or stir-fried. Limit red meat to twice a week.*

Skinless chicken or turkey breast

Fish or seafood

Vegetarian choices such as tofu, tempeh, and seitan

Lean beef such as London broil, filet mignon, and flank steak

90% lean ground beef

Veal, lamb, pork, or baked ham

**Other sides:** *During stage 1 you will not be eating starchy side dishes, because this can slow down your weight loss. In Stage 2, eat these toward the end of the meal and limit the portion size to ⅓ cup.*

Wild/brown rice

Quinoa

Barley

Whole wheat pasta

Sweet potato

## SNACKS

Plan to have a mid-morning snack and one mid-afternoon so that you do not go too long without eating. You can mix two items from the list that follows for each snack.

| Snacks | | | |
|---|---|---|---|
| Fruits | 1 cup strawberries, blueberries, blackberries, or raspberries. | | |
| | 1 cup cantaloupe, honeydew, or watermelon cubes. *Mixing berries or melons is fine, but keep the portion to 1 cup.* | | |
| | 1 small orange or grapefruit | | |
| | 1 medium apple, pear, plum, peach, or nectarine | | |
| Raw nuts and seeds | 6 to 12 almonds or cashews | | |
| | 10 to 20 peanuts | | |
| | 4 to 8 walnut halves | | |
| | 10 to 20 pistachios | | |
| | ½ ounce sunflower or pumpkin seeds | | |
| | 1 tablespoon peanut, almond, or cashew butter | | |
| Dips with crudités: *Use any combination of raw or blanched vegetables* | Carrot spears | Jícama | Serve with one of these choices: |
| | Celery sticks | Endive | |
| | Pepper slices | Radicchio | 2 to 3 tablespoons guacamole |
| | Mushrooms | Fennel | |
| | Broccoli | Zucchini | 2 to 4 tablespoons salsa |
| | Cauliflower | Asparagus | 2 to 4 tablespoons hummus |
| | Green beans | Snap peas | |
| | | Tomatoes | 2 to 4 tablespoons bean dip |
| | | Cucumbers | 2 to 4 tablespoons roasted red pepper dip |
| *Blanching, which is dropping the vegetable into boiling water for a minute and then plunging it into cold water, sets the color and makes vegetables tastier* | | | 2 tablespoons fat-free or light cream cheese |

| Snacks (*continued*) | |
| --- | --- |
| **Dairy/ Desserts** | 6 ounces low-fat plain Greek yogurt or light artificially sweetened yogurt |
| | 4 ounces plain, fat-free, or 1% fat cottage cheese or ricotta cheese |
| | 8 ounces fat-free milk, 1% milk, or unsweetened soy or almond milk |
| | 1 to 2 ounces reduced-fat cheese |
| | 1 Babybel round |
| | 1 Laughing Cow wedge |
| | 1 low-fat string cheese |
| | 4 ounces prepared fat-free, sugar-free pudding |
| | Sugar-free Popsicle or Fudgsicle |
| **Assorted** | ½ cup edamame |
| | 1 hard-boiled egg |
| | 1 cup vegetable, tomato, or lentil soup |
| | ½ avocado with 1 tablespoon simple vinaigrette |
| | 1 can sardines |
| | Lettuce wraps with 1 to 2 ounces lean deli meat (see page 153 for recipes) |
| | Protein shake or bar (see page 124–125) |

## FREE FOODS

You can eat and drink food from the following list all day long.

| Free foods | |
| --- | --- |
| Clear soup with vegetables | *We have three great recipes beginning on page 178, including one of my family's favorites.* |
| Raw vegetables | |
| Sugar-free Jell-O | |
| Coffee, tea, iced coffee, iced tea, plain or flavored seltzer, water. | *Drink plenty of water, herbal tea, seltzer, or clear soup every day. Some people eat when they are actually thirsty.* |

• • •

This chapter has given you guidelines about what to eat and what foods to avoid, along with general recommendations for what to eat for breakfast, lunch, dinner, and snacks. In the next chapter, we put all this together to give you meal plans for two weeks. The suggestions should give you ideas about all the great things you can eat and still lose weight.

# CHAPTER 8

# 14 Days of Change Your Biology Diet Meal Plans

SIMPLE, FRESH FOOD IS THE BEST WAY TO EAT. Few of my patients have time to spend hours in the kitchen preparing special foods. We have kept that in mind as we created two weeks of meal plans to get you going on the Change Your Biology Diet. We have constructed menus so that you will have leftovers you can recycle. If you follow the meal plans for two weeks, you should be able to extrapolate from them to create your own delicious meals that will fill you up, give you energy, and help to melt those pounds away. You might prefer to create your own menus from the start, which is fine. The key is to plan ahead so that you do not find yourself hungry with nothing on hand to eat. That is an easy way to backslide. You've stocked your kitchen cabinets and refrigerator with healthy food. Plan ahead so that you know what you will be eating.

## Making It Easy

There are a few kitchen items that will be a big help in preparing fresh food. A grill pan, a steamer basket, and a wok will make it a snap to prepare a meal quickly. Grilling chicken, meat, fish, vegetables, and even fruit on a grill pan on your stovetop saves time and energy. Though preparing food for a stir-fry can involve slicing and dicing, many markets now have veggies sliced and diced and ready to go. A stir-fry will cook up in a flash with a minimal amount of oil. The combinations are limitless—you can use almost anything in your refrigerator. You will find basic instructions for putting together a stir-fry on page 183. A steamer basket will help you to add more vegetables to your diet. Remember: Cooking vegetables al dente will keep you fuller longer.

Roasting a whole chicken or a turkey breast will provide you with meat for a number of meals or snacks. In a pinch, pick up a rotisserie chicken from your supermarket. Whenever you grill one boneless chicken breast, go ahead and grill several. You can use the extra chicken in many ways—sliced cold for a snack, in soups, salads, and wraps. Make big batches of soup, chili, and meat loaf, so that you can freeze individual portions for a later date. It's great to open your freezer and find it stocked with your own "convenience food." Roasted vegetables make a great side dish or snack. Crispy roasted broccoli, Brussels sprouts, kale chips, carrots, and occasionally parsnips can satisfy crunch and salt cravings.

You can eat unlimited quantities of salads filled with vegetables and fruits. Be creative. There's nothing like a kitchen sink salad in which you throw whatever you have around. Add nuts, fruit, low-fat cheese, leftover meat and/or deli meat, raw or leftover vegetables, and you have a meal.

Lettuce wraps are a terrific sandwich replacement. Fill a leaf of lettuce with a combination of hummus, any sort of cooked beans, a slice of deli meat, leftover chicken, turkey, beef, shrimp, scallops, tuna or egg salad, avocado, raw carrots, onion, pepper, spinach, any leftover cooked vegetables, salsa, guacamole, pickles, fresh herbs, or mustard. If you prefer, you can use a slice of roast beef, turkey, chicken, or ham as the outside of the wrap instead of lettuce. These constructions can be more satisfying than any standard sandwich. You won't even miss the bread.

Eggs, egg whites, and egg substitutes are so versatile. Put just

Craig, who is six feet one inch, weighed 332 pounds at his first visit. He had put on a lot of weight since his divorce. Diagnosed with sleep apnea, he had already been using a CPAP machine. I prescribed metformin and he started to eat to change his biology. What worked for him was to eat the same thing every day. Craig started with a protein shake. For lunch, he had a pound of green beans, an eight-ounce piece of salmon, and a salad. Every night for dinner, he had grilled chicken with mozzarella, tomato, tomato sauce, and more green beans. For snacks, he had slices of apples with almond butter. He told me he finds it easier to have none of something than a little of something. After a few months of eating this way, he had lost fifty-five pounds. He found himself much more energetic after losing the weight.

His biggest challenge was that when he spent time with his children, he was not able to eat his set menus. Too many choices threw Craig off. They went on vacation, and he gained five pounds. He couldn't wait to get back to his routine. We upped his metformin to twice a day. He began to run daily.

Then he added swimming three times a week. He was wearing clothing that he hadn't been able to get into for years. Craig knew it was unrealistic to expect to eat the same things every day forever, so he is making it a priority to internalize the principles of the Change Your Biology Diet, to incorporate them into his life, and to learn to trust himself to make the right food choices.

about anything into an omelet or a scramble or put a poached or fried egg on top of a bed of steamed or leftover vegetables, and you've made a balanced meal you can eat any time of day.

Think vegetables, protein, and a little fruit. This is a winning combination for weight loss and improved health. If you want to follow the meal plans to the letter, do it. If you would prefer to customize the suggested meals and snacks, that's okay, too. There is no reason to eat something you don't like. Just make sure you watch the size of your portions and remember to eat vegetables first.

## Quick Reference for Portion Sizes

| Food | Portion |
| --- | --- |
| Eggs | 1 egg = 2 egg whites = 3 tablespoons egg substitute |
| Fat-free or 2% unsweetened plain yogurt | 6 to 8 ounces |
| Fat-free or 1 to 2% cottage cheese | 6 to 8 ounces |
| Fat-free or low-fat ricotta | 6 to 8 ounces |
| Low-fat cheese | 1 to 2 ounces |
| Chicken or turkey breast | 5 ounces |
| Fish/seafood | 5 ounces |
| Beef | 5 ounces |
| Deli Meat (turkey, beef, ham) | 1 to 2 ounces |
| Extra-virgin olive oil, for cooking | 1 to 2 teaspoons |
| Salad dressing | 1 to 2 tablespoons |
| Fruit | 1 cup |
| Almonds or cashews | 6 to 12 |
| Peanuts | 10 to 20 |
| Walnuts | 4 to 8 halves |
| Pistachios | 10 to 20 |
| Sunflower or pumpkin seeds | ½ ounce |
| Almond/Peanut/Cashew Butter | 1 tablespoon |
| Guacamole | 2 to 3 tablespoons |
| Hummus | 2 to 4 tablespoons |
| Vegetables | All you can eat |

# 14 Days of Meal Plans

## Day 1

| | |
|---|---|
| Breakfast | Southwest omelet with onions, peppers, tomatoes, and salsa with two slices of turkey bacon |
| Snack | Celery with peanut or almond butter |
| Lunch | Tuna salad (made with 1 tablespoon low-fat mayonnaise, celery, onions, and fresh herbs or curry powder) on lettuce |
| Snack | Hummus with crudité |
| Dinner | Quick roast lemon chicken (page 189) with crispy roasted vegetables (on page 205)—make extra for snacks. |

## Day 2

| | |
|---|---|
| Breakfast | 2% Greek yogurt with 1 cup strawberries |
| Snack | Leftover roasted vegetables |
| Lunch | Waldorf salad with leftover quick roast lemon chicken, apples, celery, and walnuts (see pages 169–174 for dressings or use 1 tablespoon fat-free mayonnaise) |
| Snack | Low fat string cheese and almonds |
| Dinner | Grilled or baked salmon, red snapper, or cod with steamed or roasted asparagus (make extra asparagus) with balsamic vinegar and a hard-boiled egg crumbled on top |

## Day 3

| | |
|---|---|
| Breakfast | Scrambled eggs with low-fat cheese |
| Snack | Pear with nuts |

| | |
|---|---|
| Lunch | Lettuce roll-ups with hummus, asparagus, carrots, and roast beef, turkey, or ham. Or you can use the meat as the outside of the roll-up and use the lettuce inside. |
| Snack | Salsa with slices of bell pepper and carrot sticks and 1 ounce low-fat cheese |
| Dinner | Black bean soup (page 181) sprinkled with low-fat Tex-Mex mix grated cheese, chopped onion, and slices of avocado with steamed broccoli. |

### Day 4

| | |
|---|---|
| Breakfast | Diced melon with low-fat cottage cheese |
| Snack | Medium orange |
| Lunch | Turkey, chicken, veggie, or fish burger with lettuce, tomato, sliced onion, and avocado |
| Snack | Mixed nuts and low-fat cheese |
| Dinner | Mixed chopped salad, grilled or broiled steak, and cauliflower mash (page 206) |

### Day 5

| | |
|---|---|
| Breakfast | Omelet with some leftover black bean soup and a sprinkle of low-fat Tex-Mex cheese or cheddar |
| Snack | 1 cup berries |
| Lunch | Cobb salad with lettuce, sliced turkey, 1 ounce low-fat grated Swiss cheese, hard-boiled egg, avocado, and 1 piece of turkey bacon with 2 tablespoons dressing (see pages 169–174 for recipes) |

| Snack | Mixed olives with a sprinkle of extra-virgin olive oil and red pepper flakes |
| --- | --- |
| Dinner | Grilled chicken breast with oven-"fried" carrots and parsnips (see roasted vegetable recipe on page 205) and steamed broccoli with lemon |

### Day 6

| Breakfast | Protein smoothie (see recipes pages 124–125) |
| --- | --- |
| Snack | 2% Greek yogurt with shaved 70% cacao dark chocolate and sliced almonds |
| Lunch | Hearty vegetable soup (page 179) |
| Snack | Apple slices with almond or peanut butter |
| Dinner | Shrimp or chicken stir-fry with scallions, snow peas, celery, and carrot matchsticks (see stir-fry directions on page 183) |

### Day 7

| Breakfast | Low-fat cottage cheese with a sliced peach |
| --- | --- |
| Snack | Hard-boiled egg |
| Lunch | Leftover black bean soup with avocado, diced onions, and a sprinkle of low-fat cheese |
| Snack | Hummus with crudités |
| Dinner | Cup of hearty vegetable soup, beef, turkey, chicken, or fish burger, steamed green beans with almond slivers tossed with a splash of extra-virgin olive oil, and kale chips (page 205) — make extra kale chips |

## Day 8

| | |
|---|---|
| Breakfast | Poached egg on a scoop of vegetables from the vegetable soup or on a bed of steamed spinach |
| Snack | 1 ounce low-fat cheese and nuts |
| Lunch | Spinach salad with mushrooms, red onion or scallion, grated low-fat cheese, and 2 pieces of turkey bacon (see pages 169–174 for dressings) |
| Snack | Kale chips |
| Dinner | Broccoli soup (page 178), turkey piccata (page 197), or roasted turkey breast with baked zucchini (page 209) |

## Day 9

| | |
|---|---|
| Breakfast | Mushroom and spinach omelet |
| Snack | 1 cup mixed berries |
| Lunch | Black bean soup (page 181) garnished with grated cheese |
| Snack | Low-fat ricotta with scallions and chopped bell pepper |
| Dinner | Tilapia or cod with warm hot salad (page 208) |

## Day 10

| | |
|---|---|
| Breakfast | Yogurt with blueberries or 1 tablespoon slivered almonds |
| Snack | Leftover lentil salad from Day 9 |

| Lunch | Roll-ups with carrots, avocado, peppers, and sliced turkey, ham, or beef |
| --- | --- |
| Snack | Leftover broccoli soup from Day 8 |
| Dinner | Stir-fry with chicken or beef |

### Day 11

| Breakfast | Fried egg on top of a scoop of black bean soup |
| --- | --- |
| Snack | Low-fat string cheese and mixed nuts |
| Lunch | Basic chicken soup (page 175) and mixed salad |
| Snack | Celery with peanut or almond butter |
| Dinner | Turkey, chicken, or beef meat loaf (page 204) and spaghetti squash with pesto or cherry tomato sauce (page 188–189) |

### Day 12

| Breakfast | Grapefruit and mixed nuts |
| --- | --- |
| Snack | Apple slices with almond or peanut butter |
| Lunch | Leftover meat loaf with mixed salad |
| Snack | 1 cup fat-free or 1% unsweetened yogurt with 1 small diced apple, walnuts, and cinnamon |
| Dinner | Broiled or grilled chicken paillard* with arugula salad on top and a broiled or grilled tomato |

*To make a paillard, place a boneless chicken breast between two pieces of waxed paper and pound it until it is between ¼ and ½ inch thick.

## Day 13

| | |
|---|---|
| Breakfast | Diced tomatoes, cucumber, and peppers mixed with low-fat cottage cheese |
| Snack | Cup of chicken soup |
| Lunch | Chef's salad with a slice of turkey and a slice of ham, low-fat cheese, hard-boiled egg, and assorted raw vegetables |
| Snack | Sliced tomato and 1 ounce low-fat mozzarella with fresh basil and a little olive oil |
| Dinner | Shrimp cocktail and grilled lamb chop with roasted Brussels sprouts (page 205) |

## Day 14

| | |
|---|---|
| Breakfast | Scrambled eggs with diced tomato, pepper, and a sprinkle of low-fat cheese with 1 turkey, chicken, or vegetarian sausage link |
| Snack | Leftover roasted Brussels sprouts |
| Lunch | Turkey, veggie, chicken, or fish burger with onions, mushrooms, tomato, pickles, and lettuce |
| Snack | Yogurt with almonds and shaved 70% cacao dark chocolate |
| Dinner | Grilled or broiled steak, caramelized onions, and steamed spinach with sesame seeds |

# Don't Feel Like Cooking?

When you find yourself short on time or simply don't want to prepare food, you can have a frozen meal now and then. It can be a
relief not to have to be around food to prepare it when you are dieting, and your portion is automatically controlled. Since frozen meals
can contain a lot of salt and other preservatives, it is a good idea to
limit yourself to two or three a week. Try to avoid pasta, pizza, and
foods that you are not supposed to be eating, like breaded chicken,
fajitas, and any entrée with potatoes. Stick with meals that combine
protein and vegetables. In time, you will be ready to leave prepared
food behind in favor of delicious fresh food. These are the guidelines
I recommend when you select a frozen meal:

- 250 to 300 calories
- Less than 10 grams of fat
- Less than 40 grams of carbohydrates
- More than 3 grams of fiber
- More than 15 grams of protein

It's a good idea to make a simple side salad to begin the meal to
make you feel more full and satisfied.

•  •  •

The recipes in the next chapter will give you ideas for "dressing up"
the food you eat. You will see that you do not have to be stuck eating
boring food that tastes like sawdust just because you are trying to
lose weight.

# CHAPTER 9

# Quick, Easy, and Delicious Recipes

CHANGING THE WAY YOU EAT does not mean you can't eat well. The recipes in this chapter should convince you there is a world of wonderful food available to you when you are eating to change your biology. To help you expand your repertoire for preparing the protein and vegetables you will be focusing on, we have collected recipes for colorful and sophisticated dishes that will make you forget you are on a diet. The food is so tasty, your family and friends will enjoy eating what you do. The healthy dips and spreads prove that you can snack on a lot more than hummus, though there is nothing wrong with hummus. The salad dressings will make your salads a treat, and you will want to keep individual portions of the meal-worthy soups in your freezer. There are general guidelines for building a stir-fry—a great way to "toss" a meal together. We concentrated on sauces for your grilled, poached, broiled, and steamed chicken, fish, beef, and vegetables that are caloric bargains. Since you will be eating a lot of chicken and fish, we have provided recipes that demonstrate that eating plain grilled meat and steamed vegetables is a choice, not a necessity. With a little planning and only a bit more time, you will be turning out gourmet meals that will fill you up and make you happy. Enjoy!

# Breakfast/All-Day Snack

You know how important it is to start the day with protein. You can make delicious omelets in advance with the recipe that follows—no muss, no fuss.

## Cheese and Veggie "Cupcake" Omelets

*Makes 6 servings, 2 omelets per serving*

If making yourself an omelet in the morning is not going to happen, these "cupcake" omelets are the answer. You can make a full muffin pan of them and refrigerate or freeze what you do not eat. Having a supply in the refrigerator or freezer will insure you have a quick, high-protein breakfast on hand. Just warm up two omelets in the microwave and you are good to go. These protein-dense "cupcakes" are terrific as a snack, too.

> 4 cups broccoli florets, torn spinach, inch-long pieces
>     asparagus, sliced mushrooms, diced peppers, or diced
>     onions (use any vegetable or combination)
> 1 teaspoon extra-virgin olive oil
> Sea salt and freshly ground black pepper
> 5 large eggs
> 1 cup egg whites
> ¼ cup grated low-fat Parmesan cheese (optional)
> ¼ cup reduced-fat shredded cheddar, Swiss, Colby, or
>     Monterey Jack cheese

1. Preheat the oven to 350°F.
2. Steam the vegetable(s) of your choice for about 6 minutes.
3. Transfer the vegetable(s) to a bowl and add the olive oil and salt and pepper to taste. Toss to combine.
4. Line a 12-cup muffin tin with paper liners or spray the pan with cooking spray. Divide the vegetables evenly among the wells of the pan.

5. Whisk together the eggs, egg whites, grated Parmesan, and salt and pepper to taste in a medium bowl. Pour the egg mixture over the vegetables in each well until they are three-quarters full. Top with the shredded cheese and bake for about 20 minutes.

# Spreads and Dips

You do not have to sacrifice flavor to lose weight. Spreads and dips are a great way to spice up your diet and satisfy your crunch craving. You can snack on them with raw vegetables, season your eggs with them, use them as a dipping sauce for chicken, fish, or beef, or as a spread on your roll-ups. Hummus is the go-to dip on the meal plans, but you can have any one of the recipes that follow instead. You will make a habit of keeping chopped up, raw vegetables in your refrigerator when you know you'll be putting them to good use.

## Avocado Yogurt Dip with a Kick

*Makes 16 servings, 2 tablespoons per serving*

This creamy dip can be prepared 8 hours in advance and refrigerated in an airtight container.

> 3 ripe avocados, pitted, peeled, and coarsely chopped
> ¾ cup fat-free Greek yogurt
> ½ cup chopped red onion
> 3 tablespoons chopped fresh cilantro
> 2 tablespoons fresh lime juice
> 1 tablespoon seeded chopped jalapeño pepper
> 1 tablespoon ground cumin
> 1 garlic clove, minced
> ½ teaspoon sea salt

1. Combine all the ingredients in a food processor or blender and process until smooth.

## Mediterranean Bean Dip

*Makes 8 servings, 2 tablespoons per serving*

This satisfying dip is heart healthy and provides extra protein.

    1 (16-ounce) can cannellini beans, drained and rinsed
    1 (7-ounce) jar roasted red bell peppers, drained and rinsed
    ¼ cup chopped fresh basil
    1 garlic clove
    1 teaspoon balsamic vinegar
    2 tablespoons extra-virgin olive oil
    ½ teaspoon sea salt
    ½ teaspoon freshly ground black pepper

1.  Combine the beans, roasted peppers, basil, garlic, and vinegar in a food processor or blender and process until smooth.
2.  Slowly add the olive oil through the feed tube with the processor running. Stir in the salt and black pepper.

## Cool Dip

*Makes 8 servings, 2 tablespoons per serving*

This refreshing cucumber and dill dip is very versatile. It's great with raw vegetables, can be used instead of mayonnaise on a wrap, and makes a delicious sauce for fish, especially salmon.

    1 cup grated English (seedless) cucumber
    ½ cup fat-free Greek yogurt
    ½ cup light sour cream
    3 tablespoons chopped fresh dill
    1 teaspoon grated garlic
    ¼ teaspoon sea salt
    ¼ teaspoon freshly ground black pepper
    Sliced cucumber, for garnish

1.  Combine all the ingredients except the sliced cucumber in a bowl and mix together. Garnish with cucumber slices.

## Nutty Edamame Spread
*Makes 16 servings, 2 tablespoons per serving*

2 cups frozen shelled edamame
2 garlic cloves
½ cup packed fresh basil leaves
2 tablespoons pine nuts, toasted
2 tablespoons 2% Greek yogurt
¼ cup water
2 tablespoons extra-virgin olive oil
2 tablespoons fresh lemon juice
¾ teaspoon sea salt
½ teaspoon grated lemon zest
Freshly ground black pepper
Strips of lemon zest, for garnish

1.  In a small saucepan, combine the edamame and garlic and add water to cover the edamame by 2 inches.
2.  Bring to a boil and cook until the edamame is tender, about 2 minutes. Remove from the heat and drain.
3.  Transfer the edamame and garlic to a food processer and add the basil, pine nuts, and yogurt. Pulse until coarsely ground, about 10 pulses.
4.  Add the water, olive oil, lemon juice, salt, and lemon zest and process until almost smooth. Season with pepper.
5.  Garnish with lemon zest strips.

## Sun-Dried Tomato and White Bean Dip

*Makes 8 servings, 2 tablespoons per serving*

1 head garlic
1 cup water
1 (3.5-ounce) package sun-dried tomatoes without oil
1 (15.8-ounce) can great northern beans, drained and rinsed
1 tablespoon extra-virgin olive oil
½ teaspoon chopped fresh rosemary
¼ teaspoon sea salt
Freshly ground black pepper

1. Preheat the oven to 375°F.
2. Remove the outer white papery skin from the garlic head. Wrap the head in aluminum foil. Bake for 45 minutes, then let cool for 10 minutes.
3. Separate the cloves and squeeze out the garlic pulp. Toss out the skins.
4. In a saucepan, bring the water to a boil. Add the tomatoes, then cover the pan and remove from the heat. Let the tomatoes stand for 10 minutes.
5. Drain the tomatoes in a sieve over a bowl and reserve ¼ cup of the liquid.
6. Transfer the roasted garlic, tomatoes, and reserved soaking liquid to a food processor. Add the remaining ingredients and pepper to taste and process until smooth.

## Olive-Mustard Tapenade

*Makes 8 servings, 2 tablespoons per serving*

This tart Mediterranean tapenade is great with poultry, fish, and vegetables, and in wraps. This keeps well, covered, in the refrigerator. You should have some on hand to use as a flavor booster.

¼ cup chopped pitted Kalamata olives
¼ cup chopped pitted green olives
1 tablespoon chopped fresh parsley
1 tablespoon Dijon mustard
2 teaspoons balsamic vinegar
½ teaspoon minced fresh garlic or granulated garlic

1. In a bowl, combine all the ingredients.

# Salad Dressings

Homemade salad dressings are so much tastier than store-bought ones, which are usually loaded with chemicals anyway. Since you will be eating a lot of salads to change your biology, making a good salad dressing is well worth your while. You can experiment with different vinegars and infused oils. A simple vinaigrette made with excellent extra-virgin olive oil and vinegar or lemon in a ratio of 3 or 4 to 1, a teaspoon of Dijon mustard, and salt and pepper is perfection. Just shake it up in a jar with a lid. The recipes that follow go beyond the classics and give you high-flavor dressings that will not put you over the top in calorie consumption.

## Champagne Vinaigrette
*Makes 10 servings, 2 tablespoons per serving*

This is a light and delicate dressing. Mixing the ingredients in a blender creates a creamy consistency. If you prefer, you can mince the shallot and whisk the ingredients together in a bowl.

1 shallot, quartered
¼ cup champagne vinegar
¼ cup extra-virgin olive oil
1 tablespoon Dijon mustard
½ teaspoon sea salt
Freshly ground black pepper

1.  Combine all the ingredients in a blender and puree until
    smooth.

......................................................................................

## Zesty Lemon-Mint Vinaigrette

*Makes 12 servings, 2 tablespoons per serving*

This dressing sparkles with the flavor of cool mint and tart
lemon. It enhances steamed vegetables and makes a salad come
alive.

> ⅓ cup fresh lemon juice
> 1 tablespoon Dijon mustard
> 1 teaspoon sugar substitute, preferably stevia
> 1 garlic clove, minced
> ⅓ cup extra-virgin olive oil
> ⅓ cup chopped fresh mint
> Pinch of sea salt
> Freshly ground black pepper

1.  In a small bowl, whisk together the lemon juice, mustard,
    sugar substitute, and garlic until blended.
2.  While whisking, drizzle in the oil until emulsified.
3.  Stir in the mint, salt, and pepper to taste.

......................................................................................

## Simple Asian Vinaigrette

*Makes 4 servings, 2 tablespoons per serving*

This is a delicate dressing to use whenever you want to add
Asian flair.

> ½ small garlic clove, finely grated
> 1 tablespoon reduced-sodium soy sauce
> 2 teaspoons unseasoned rice vinegar
> ⅓ cup extra-virgin olive oil

½ teaspoon toasted sesame oil
Sea salt and freshly ground black pepper

1. In a small bowl, whisk together the garlic, soy sauce, and vinegar.
2. Gradually whisk in the olive oil, then the sesame oil. The dressing will thicken slightly. Season with salt and pepper.
3. Transfer to a jar, cover, and chill until use.

## Herbed Cucumber Vinaigrette

*Makes 10 servings, 2 tablespoons per serving*

This dressing has a luxurious texture because vegetables are pureed into the dressing, giving it body.

1 small cucumber, peeled, seeded, and chopped
¼ cup extra-virgin olive oil
2 tablespoons red-wine vinegar
2 tablespoons chopped fresh chives
2 tablespoons chopped fresh parsley
1 tablespoon fat-free Greek yogurt
1 teaspoon Dijon mustard
1 teaspoon prepared horseradish
1 packet sugar substitute, preferably stevia
½ teaspoon sea salt

1. Combine all the ingredients in a blender and puree until smooth.

## Low-Calorie Creamy Caesar

*Makes 8 servings, 2 tablespoons per serving*

When you crave a salad with Caesar dressing, treat yourself to this low-calorie version. It will not disappoint.

⅓ cup fat-free Greek yogurt
2 tablespoons lemon juice
1 tablespoon extra-virgin olive oil
1 garlic clove, minced
2 teaspoons red wine vinegar
2 teaspoons Worcestershire sauce
1 teaspoon anchovy paste (optional)
1 teaspoon Dijon mustard
½ teaspoon freshly ground black pepper

1. Combine all the ingredients in a jar with a lid, cover, and shake to blend.

## Greek Island Dressing

*Makes 8 servings, 2 tablespoons per serving*

A salad dressed with Greek Island Dressing is an excellent side for grilled fish. You can imagine you are sitting at a café in the warm sun on an idyllic Greek island.

¼ cup extra-virgin olive oil
¼ cup low-sodium chicken stock
¼ cup fresh lemon juice
¼ cup red wine vinegar
1 garlic clove, minced
1 teaspoon dried oregano
¼ teaspoon freshly ground black pepper

1. Combine all the ingredients in a jar with a lid, cover, and shake to blend. Let the dressing sit at room temperature for 1 or 2 hours so that the flavors blend.

## Green Goddess Dressing

*Makes 6 servings, 2 tablespoons per serving*

This is the classic, with almost all the calories gone.

¼ cup low-fat cottage cheese
3 tablespoons buttermilk
1 tablespoon chopped fresh parsley
1 or 2 garlic cloves, minced
1½ teaspoons apple cider vinegar
⅛ teaspoon hot sauce
Pinch of sea salt

1. Combine all the ingredients in a blender and blend until smooth.

## Creamy Dill Ranch

*Makes 10 servings, 2 tablespoons per serving*

If you are missing creamy dressings, this is a delicious low-calorie substitute. It's very rich.

1 small shallot
¾ cup fat-free cottage cheese
¼ cup reduced-fat mayonnaise
2 tablespoons buttermilk powder (can be found in baking
    section with the powdered milk)
2 tablespoons white wine vinegar
¼ cup skim milk
1 tablespoon chopped fresh dill
¼ teaspoon sea salt
¼ teaspoon freshly ground black pepper

1. With the food processor running, pass the shallot through the feed tube and process until finely chopped.

2. Add the cottage cheese, mayonnaise, buttermilk powder, and vinegar. Process until smooth.
3. Pour in the milk while the processor is running.
4. Scrape down the sides of the processor bowl, add the dill, salt, and pepper, and process until combined.

## Creamy Curry Dressing

*Makes 5 servings, 2 tablespoons per serving*

This exotic dressing will bring a new dimension to salads or vegetables.

½ cup fat-free Greek yogurt
½ cup low-fat mayonnaise
3 tablespoons fresh lemon juice
2 tablespoons water
1 tablespoon sugar substitute
1 teaspoon curry powder
Sea salt and freshly ground black pepper

1. Combine all the ingredients in a blender and blend until smooth, or whisk together in a small bowl.

# Soups

When deciding on soups to include in this section, we wanted to give you some hearty soups that would fill you up. Some of the recipes are closer to stews than simple soups. With a mixed green salad, each of these soups makes a perfect meal. It's always a gift to have leftover soup, because you can freeze it for another day. Having your freezer stocked with individual portions of soup is a blessing when you just don't feel like cooking. You can sip clear or vegetable soups all day.

# Basic Chicken Soup from Scratch

*Makes 6 servings, 1½ cups per serving*

Chicken soup is the ultimate comfort food. This soup is a great base. You can add some steamed vegetables at the last few minutes, cooked quinoa when you are eating carbohydrates, and all sorts of herbs. Dill is a fragrant and tasty addition.

> 1 (3½- to 4-pound) chicken
> 6 carrots
> 4 celery stalks
> 1 large yellow onion, quartered
> 1½ teaspoons sea salt
> 1 teaspoon whole black peppercorns

1. Place the chicken in a large pot.
2. Cut 3 of the carrots and 2 of the celery stalks into 1-inch pieces and add them to the pot with the chicken. Add the onion, salt, peppercorns, and enough cold water to cover (about 8 cups).
3. Bring the water to a boil. Reduce the heat to maintain a simmer and cook, skimming any foam that rises to the top, until the chicken is cooked through, about 30 minutes.
4. Transfer the chicken to a bowl and let cool.
5. Strain the broth and discard the vegetables. Return the broth to the pot.
6. Thinly slice the remaining carrots and celery. Add them to the broth and simmer until tender, about 10 minutes.
7. When the chicken is cool enough to handle, shred the meat and add it to the soup.

# Chicken and Spinach Soup with Pesto

*Makes 5 servings, 1½ cups per serving*

This satisfying soup takes only thirty minutes to make. You do not have to make fresh pesto. Instead, you can substitute 3 or 4 tablespoons store-bought pesto.

> 2 teaspoons extra-virgin olive oil
> 8 ounces boneless, skinless chicken breast, quartered
> ¼ cup sliced carrots
> ¼ cup diced red bell pepper
> 1 garlic clove, minced
> 5 cups low-sodium chicken broth
> 1½ teaspoons dried marjoram
> 1 (15-ounce) can great northern or cannellini beans, drained
>     and rinsed
> 6 ounces baby spinach, coarsely chopped

For the fresh pesto (optional):

> 1 tablespoon extra-virgin olive oil
> ⅓ cup fresh basil leaves
> ¼ cup grated Parmesan cheese
> Fresh ground black pepper

1. Heat the oil in a Dutch oven or a large saucepan over medium-high heat.
2. Add the chicken, carrots, and bell pepper and cook, stirring frequently, until the chicken begins to brown, 3 to 4 minutes. Add the garlic and stir for 1 minute more.
3. Stir in the broth and marjoram and bring to a boil over high heat. Reduce the heat to maintain a simmer and cook until the chicken is cooked through, about 5 minutes.
4. Transfer the chicken to a cutting board with a slotted spoon and let cool.
5. Add the beans and spinach to the pot and bring to a boil. Cook for 5 minutes.
6. To make the fresh pesto, combine the oil, basil, and Parme-

san in a food processor. Process to a coarse paste, add a little water, and scrape down the sides.

7.  Cut the chicken into bite-size pieces. Stir the chicken and pesto into the pot.

8.  Season with pepper.

## Sweet-and-Sour Beef Soup

*Makes 6 servings, 1¾ cups per serving*

This fragrant soup is more like a flavorful stew. It's great on a rainy or cold day.

> 1 tablespoon extra-virgin olive oil
> 1 pound 90% lean ground beef
> 1½ teaspoons caraway seeds
> 1 teaspoon dried thyme
> 1¼ cups chopped bell pepper
> 1¼ cups chopped onion
> 1 medium sweet-tart cooking apple, such as Cortland,
>   Yellow Delicious, or Ida Red, unpeeled, cored, and diced
> 6 cups low-sodium beef broth
> 1 (15-ounce) can crushed tomatoes
> 1 packet sugar substitute
> 1 tablespoon Hungarian sweet paprika
> 3 cups coarsely chopped savoy or green cabbage
> 2 tablespoons apple cider vinegar
> ¼ teaspoon sea salt
> Freshly ground black pepper

1.  Heat the oil in a Dutch oven over medium heat. Add the beef, caraway, and thyme and cook, stirring and breaking up the beef with a spoon, until the beef has browned, about 4 minutes.

2.  Stir in the bell pepper, onion, and apple. Cook, stirring, for 2 to 3 minutes.

3.  Stir in the broth, tomatoes, sugar substitute, and paprika and bring the mixture to a boil. Cook for 8 to 10 minutes.
4.  Stir in the cabbage and cook until just tender, 3 to 4 minutes.
5.  Season with the vinegar, salt, and pepper to taste.

## Broccoli Soup

*Makes 6 servings, 1 cup per serving*

I guarantee that this is a terrific soup. It's a family favorite. Our kids always ask for it at holiday time. It's based on a Martha Stewart recipe, but my wife, Jane, leaves out the butter, cream, and salt.

  1½ tablespoons extra-virgin olive oil
  8 carrots, minced
  4 leeks (white parts only), minced
  4 garlic cloves, minced
  6 cups low-sodium chicken broth
  1 head broccoli, cut into small florets (6 to 8 cups)
  ½ teaspoon celery seed
  Pinch of cayenne pepper

1.  In a pot, warm the olive oil over medium heat.
2.  Add the carrots, leeks, and garlic. Cook until tender, 6 to 8 minutes. Do not brown.
3.  Add the broth and bring it to a simmer.
4.  Add the broccoli and simmer until the broccoli is tender, 15 to 20 minutes.
5.  Carefully pour the soup into a food processor and process until the veggies are chopped but not pureed.
6.  Pour the soup back into the pot. Stir in the celery seed and cayenne pepper.
7.  Reheat before serving.

## EZ Vegetable Soup

*Makes 10 servings, 1 cup per serving*

You can have a cup of this soup whenever you are hungry. Make a double batch and freeze some. This soup can become your go-to snack.

> 1 teaspoon extra-virgin olive oil
> 1 large yellow onion, chopped
> 3 garlic cloves, chopped
> 8 cups low-sodium vegetable or chicken broth
> 2 medium bell peppers — make it colorful with red, orange, or yellow or a combo
> 2 cups small broccoli florets
> 2 cups baby carrots, halved crosswise
> 1 cup green beans, halved
> ½ cup thinly sliced celery
> Sea salt and freshly ground black pepper

1. In a large pot, heat the oil over medium-high heat.
2. Add the onion and garlic and cook, stirring, until golden, about 3 minutes.
3. Add the broth and vegetables and bring to a boil.
4. Simmer until the vegetables are tender, about 30 minutes. Add sea salt and pepper to taste.

## Hearty Vegetable Soup

*Makes 10 servings, 1½ cups per serving*

This is a remarkably versatile soup. You can get many meals out of it. If you remove some vegetables with a slotted spoon, you can use them in an omelet or a wrap. If you want to make the soup even heartier, add shredded chicken breast, some rotisserie chicken, or a piece of firm fish like haddock. This soup freezes well.

2 tablespoons extra-virgin olive oil
1 large carrot, thinly sliced
1 medium parsnip, thinly sliced
2 leeks, thinly sliced
½ small onion, thinly sliced
1 celery stalk, thinly sliced
2 garlic cloves, diced
1 cup chopped kale
1 cup chopped collard greens
1 cup shredded cabbage
2 (15-ounce) cans organic great northern beans
     (or any kind), drained and rinsed
1½ cups diced tomatoes with their juices
1 quart vegetable broth or water
1 teaspoon thyme
Whole bay leaf

1. In a large Dutch oven or stockpot, heat the olive oil over medium-high heat.
2. Add the carrot, parsnip, leeks, onion, celery, and garlic and cook, stirring, until softened.
3. Add the kale, collard greens, and cabbage and stir to coat.
4. Reduce the heat to low and cover the pot. Cook until the greens are wilted and soft, about 3 minutes.
5. Add the beans and tomatoes with their juices. Increase the heat to bring the soup up to a simmer.
6. Add the broth and bring the soup back up to a simmer. Add the thyme and bay leaf. Simmer for at least 30 minutes.

## White Bean, Escarole, and Chicken Sausage Soup
*Makes 4 servings, 1½ cups per serving*

What is great about this recipe, besides that it tastes so good, is that it is quick to make. You can throw it together in 15 minutes.

½ pound cooked chicken sausages, sliced
2 tablespoons extra-virgin olive oil
2 garlic cloves, sliced
6 cups low-sodium chicken broth
1 (15.5-ounce) can cannellini beans, drained and rinsed
1 small head escarole, torn
½ teaspoon sea salt
¼ teaspoon freshly ground black pepper

1. In a large pot, cook the sausages in the oil over medium-high heat until browned, 3 to 5 minutes.
2. Add the garlic and cook, stirring, for 1 minute.
3. Add the chicken broth, beans, escarole, salt, and pepper. Simmer until the escarole is tender, 8 to 10 minutes.

## Black Bean Soup

*Makes 4 servings, 1 cup per serving*

Black bean soup sticks to your ribs. Dress it up with chopped onions, tomatoes, and avocados. You can use a dollop of this thick, tasty soup to spice up a wrap or in an omelet.

1 tablespoon extra-virgin olive oil
1 medium onion, chopped
12 garlic cloves, minced
2 (15-ounce) cans black beans, drained and rinsed
1¾ cups vegetable broth
2 teaspoons chili powder
1 teaspoon ground cumin
½ cup fresh chopped cilantro
Avocado, pitted, peeled, and diced (optional)
1 lime, cut into wedges

1. In a 3-quart pot, heat the oil over medium heat. Add the onion and garlic and cook until tender.

2. Stir in the beans, broth, chili powder, and cumin and bring to a boil.
3. Reduce the heat to low and simmer for 15 minutes.
4. Use a blender, food processor, or a counter mixer to blend the soup to a creamy consistency.
5. Garnish with the cilantro, avocado, if desired, and lime wedges.

## Shrimp and Scallop Stew

*Makes 2 servings, 1¾ cups per serving*

Stewing seafood is a traditional way to prepare fish and shell-fish. It keeps the seafood tender and sweet and creates a wonderful broth.

> 2 tablespoons extra-virgin olive oil
> 1 medium onion, chopped
> 1 garlic clove, minced
> ½ teaspoon dried thyme
> ½ teaspoon fennel seed
> ¼ teaspoon sea salt
> ¼ teaspoon freshly ground black pepper
> Pinch of saffron threads, crumbled
> 1 cup diced tomatoes with their juices (can be canned)
> ¼ cup vegetable broth
> ¼ pound green beans, cut into 1-inch pieces
> ¼ pound bay scallops
> ¼ pound small shrimp, peeled and deveined

1. In a large saucepan, heat the oil over medium heat. Add the onion and cook, stirring, for 3 minutes.
2. Add the garlic, thyme, fennel seed, salt, pepper, and saffron and cook for 30 seconds.

3. Stir in the tomatoes with their juices, broth, and beans. Bring to a simmer. Cover and reduce the heat. Simmer for 2 minutes.

4. Raise the heat to medium, stir in the scallops, and cook for 2 minutes.

5. Add the shrimp and cook for 2 minutes more, stirring occasionally.

## How to Build a Stir Fry

*1 serving*

Mastering the art of stir-frying will enable you to whip up a meal in no time.

Making a stir fry is quick and easy, especially if you have leftover meat. All it takes is five quick steps:

| Step | Item | Instructions |
|------|------|--------------|
| 1 | 1 tablespoon canola oil | Heat a wok over medium-high heat and add canola oil. |
| 2 | Vegetables (pick two):<br>1 cup whole snap peas<br>1 cup thinly sliced Napa cabbage<br>1 cup sliced mushrooms<br>1 cup blanched baby bok choy<br>½ cup chopped bell pepper<br>½ cup blanched broccoli<br>½ cup green beans, cut and blanched<br>½ cup peas<br>½ cup thinly sliced onion<br>⅓ cup carrots, thinly sliced<br>2 tablespoons shelled edamame | Add the vegetables and stir-fry for 1 minute. |

| Step | Item | Instructions (continued) |
|------|------|--------------------------|
| 3 | **Protein (pick one):** <br><br> 4 ounces sautéed extra firm tofu <br><br> 3½ ounces steamed shrimp <br><br> 2 ounces roasted or poached chicken <br><br> 2 ounces lean sautéed flank steak | Add the cooked protein, let it sizzle for 30 seconds, then stir-fry for 30 seconds more, or until done. |
| 4 | **Sauce (pick one or two):** <br><br> Low sodium soy sauce <br><br> Beef, chicken or vegetable broth <br><br> Sesame oil <br><br> Rice vinegar <br><br> Bottled hoisin <br><br> Sesame garlic <br><br> General Tso <br><br> Sriracha sauce. | Add the sauce or flavoring. |
| 5 | **Crunch on top (pick one or any combination):** <br><br> ½ cup thinly sliced scallions <br><br> ½ cup bean sprouts <br><br> ½ cup thinly sliced daikon radish <br><br> A sprinkling of sesame seeds, nuts, or crushed red pepper | Finish with something crunchy. |

# Sauces

If you get tired of plain steamed vegetables and grilled chicken or fish, you can make a simple, low-calorie sauce to break the monotony and make your food more varied. To lose weight, the food you eat does not have to be bland. We've pulled together some sauces that will enliven your food without making you stray from the program.

## Butterless White Wine Sauce

*Makes 6 servings, 1½ tablespoons per serving*

This twist on a classic white wine sauce will do the trick without being fattening.

⅓ cup chopped onion
½ cup low-sodium chicken broth
¼ cup dry white wine
2 tablespoons white wine vinegar
2 tablespoons extra-virgin olive oil
2 teaspoons chopped fresh chives

1. Heat a skillet over medium high heat and coat with cooking spray.
2. Add the onion to the pan and cook, stirring, for 2 minutes.
3. Add the chicken broth, wine, and vinegar and bring to a boil. Cook until the liquid has reduced to ¼ cup, about 5 minutes.
4. Remove from the heat and stir in the oil and fresh chives.

## Garlicky Chickpea Sauce

*Makes 9 servings, 1½ tablespoons per serving*

This rustic Italian sauce is creamy. It can be used on veggies or chicken or as a pasta sauce when you are eating carbs.

2 teaspoons extra-virgin olive oil
4 garlic cloves: 2 crushed, 2 minced
14 ounces low-sodium chicken broth
1 (15-ounce) can chickpeas, drained and rinsed

¾ teaspoon sea salt
¼ teaspoon red pepper flakes
1 tablespoon minced fresh parsley
1 tablespoon fresh lemon juice

1.  In a medium saucepan, heat the oil over medium heat.
2.  Add the crushed garlic and cook, stirring, for 1 minute.
3.  Add the broth, chickpeas, salt, and red pepper flakes and bring to a boil. Cover, reduce the heat, and simmer for 15 minutes.
4.  Transfer the chickpea mixture to a food processor and process until smooth.
5.  Stir in the minced garlic, parsley, and lemon juice.

## Chimichurri Sauce

*Makes 8 servings, 1 tablespoon per serving*

This Argentinian pesto, used on grilled meat, is a caloric bargain with big flavor. This recipe reduces the amount of oil usually used.

1 cup lightly packed fresh parsley leaves
½ cup water
¼ cup red-wine vinegar
¼ cup extra-virgin olive oil
2 large garlic cloves, smashed
1 teaspoon dried thyme
¼ teaspoon red pepper flakes
½ teaspoon sea salt
Freshly ground black pepper

1.  Combine all the ingredients in a blender or food processor and blend until coarsely chopped.

# Fresh Vegetable Sauce

*Makes 4 servings, 1 cup per serving*

This sauce is full of healthy vegetables. Eaten with chicken, fish, or beef, it makes a meal. You might want a salad for extra crunch.

1 eggplant
1 teaspoon sea salt, plus more for the eggplant
1 onion, diced
2 to 3 tablespoons water
2 summer squash, diced
1 red bell pepper, chopped
1 green bell pepper, chopped
4 garlic cloves, minced
1 (28 ounce) can fire-roasted tomatoes
1 tablespoon tomato paste
1½ teaspoons dried oregano
Freshly ground black pepper
¼ cup packed fresh basil

1.  Peel the eggplant and cut it into ½-inch slices. Lay the slices in a large colander in a single layer and lightly salt them. Turn them over and salt the other side. Put the colander on a plate and set it aside for about a half hour.
2.  After 30 minutes, rinse the eggplant and chop it into ½-inch cubes.
3.  Heat a large nonstick saucepan and add the onion and 2 tablespoons of the water. Cook, stirring, until the onion begins to brown.
4.  Add the eggplant and a little more water. Continue to cook, stirring occasionally, until the eggplant is mostly cooked, about 8 minutes.
5.  Add the squash, bell peppers, and garlic, and continue to cook and stir for 3 minutes more.
6.  Add the remaining ingredients, except for the fresh basil.

Cover and cook over low heat until all the flavors have blended, about 10 minutes.

7.  Add the basil and cook for a couple minutes more.

## Herbed Mustard Sauce

*Makes 4 servings, 1½ tablespoons per serving*

Tangy mustard sauce without the cream is a dream come true. Enjoy this sauce on everything.

½ cup Dijon mustard
3 tablespoons chopped fresh dill
3 tablespoons chopped fresh basil
2 tablespoons fresh lemon juice
1 teaspoon extra-virgin olive oil

1.  Combine all the ingredients in a medium bowl and stir together.

## Cherry Tomato Sauce

*Makes 8 servings, 2 tablespoons per serving*

This quick, colorful sauce is good with just about anything. Try it on spaghetti squash when you have a pasta craving. Use multicolored cherry tomatoes for eye appeal.

3 tablespoons extra-virgin olive oil
3 garlic cloves, crushed
½ cup diced eggplant, bell pepper, onion, summer squash,
    or anchovies for flavor, or a mixture of any of these
    ingredients
1 pint cherry tomatoes, halved
1 tablespoon dried rosemary or dried oregano
Sea salt and freshly ground black pepper
Fresh basil or parsley, for garnish

1. In a 10- or 11-inch skillet, heat the olive oil and garlic gently over low heat—let the garlic soften, not brown.
2. Turn up the heat and add the diced vegetables (or anchovy) you are using for flavor and cook until they are soft.
3. Add the cherry tomatoes, rosemary, and salt and pepper to taste.
4. Turn up the heat and simmer until the sauce is thick and pulpy, 15 to 20 minutes.
5. Remove the saucepan from the heat and stir in the basil.

# Chicken and Turkey

Since you will be eating a lot of chicken, we have put together recipes that will show you just how much you can do with one of the staples of your diet.

## Quick Roast Lemon Chicken

*Serves 4 to 6*

This is a perfect recipe, which has been adapted from one originally by Marcella Hazan, a great Italian cook. It has become so popular that everyone roasts chicken this way. The recipe produces a perfect chicken every time, and you'll have leftovers to recycle in another meal. Use this simple recipe when you are in a rush because it calls for a small broiler, which cooks quickly. You could even roast two chickens at once.

1 small broiler chicken (2½ pounds)
Sea salt and freshly ground black pepper
Hot sauce (optional)
2 lemons

1. Preheat the oven to 350°F.
2. Wash the chicken inside and out. Pat it dry.

3. Sprinkle the salt and pepper—inside and out—and rub the seasoning into the surfaces of the chicken with your fingertips. Sprinkle some hot sauce on the skin, if desired.

4. Wash the lemons and soften them up by pressing them between your palms and rolling them back and forth a few times.

5. Pierce the lemons with a fork and place them inside the chicken. You can close the cavity opening with toothpicks if you like, but it's not necessary.

6. Put the roasting pan in the upper third of the oven and roast for 35 minutes.

7. Turn up the oven temperature to 400°F and roast for 15 minutes more. If you're lucky, the skin will puff up.

8. Remove and discard the lemons. Let sit for 5 minutes before slicing.

## Poached Chicken and Vegetables

*Serves 4*

This colorful dish has a terrific combination of vegetables and textures. It's a great way to increase your vegetable consumption.

> 1 cup low-sodium chicken broth
> 1 cup cauliflower florets
> 1 cup sliced green beans
> 1 cup diced red bell pepper
> 1 cup fresh or frozen peas
> 1 cup frozen pearl onions
> ½ cup water
> 1¼ pounds skinless, boneless chicken breasts, cut into
>     1-inch cubes
> 1 tablespoon fresh lemon juice
> Freshly ground black pepper
> 8 large iceberg lettuce leaves

1. Combine the broth, vegetables, and water in a large frying pan.
2. Arrange the chicken over the vegetables. Sprinkle the chicken with the lemon juice and pepper to taste. Cover with the lettuce.
3. Bring to a boil, then reduce the heat to low and cook, covered, until the chicken is tender, about 25 minutes.
4. Discard the lettuce and drain the liquid from the pan. Arrange the vegetables with the chicken on a platter.

## Chicken Breast with Asparagus and Carrots in a Parchment Packet
*Serves 4*

A gourmet would call this method *en papillote*, which means "in parchment." Parchment packets are often used in traditional French cooking.

> 4 boneless, skinless chicken breasts, cut crosswise
>     into ¼-inch strips
> ¼ teaspoon sea salt, plus more to taste
> Freshly ground black pepper
> ½ pound asparagus, cut into 1-inch lengths
> 1 medium onion, thinly sliced
> 1 medium carrot, cut into julienne strips
> 2 tablespoons extra-virgin olive oil
> 2 teaspoons fresh lemon juice
> Dash of cayenne pepper
> 4 tablespoons dried tarragon

1. Preheat the oven to 450°F.
2. Tear off four lengths of parchment paper or heavy-duty aluminum foil large enough to wrap the chicken and vegetables and allow for heat circulation and expansion, about 12 x 18 inches.

3. Place the sliced chicken in the center of the lower half of each length of paper or foil. Season with salt and pepper. Top with the asparagus, onion, and carrot.

4. Combine the extra-virgin olive oil, lemon juice, ¼ teaspoon salt, and cayenne in a small bowl. Pour equally over each chicken-vegetable serving. Sprinkle 1 tablespoon of dried tarragon on each serving.

5. Fold the upper half of the paper or foil over the ingredients, making a series of locked folds. Repeat the folds for ends, pressing tight to seal.

6. Place the packets in a single layer on a baking sheet. Cook for 18 to 20 minutes, until the chicken is cooked through.

7. To serve, cut an X in the top of each packet (be careful — the steam will be hot) and fold the parchment or foil back and serve on individual plates, or transfer the contents of the packets to individual plates.

## Chicken Florentine with Mushrooms

*Serves 4*

The combination of flavors in this dish is memorable, and it looks great, too.

4 boneless, skinless chicken breasts
1 small onion, quartered
1 tablespoon extra-virgin olive oil
2 cups sliced mushrooms
2 cups chopped cooked fresh spinach, or 1 (10-ounce)
     package frozen chopped spinach, cooked and drained
¼ teaspoon ground nutmeg
¼ teaspoon sea salt
Freshly ground black pepper
4 teaspoons grated low-fat Parmesan cheese

1. Preheat the broiler.

2. In a medium saucepan, combine the chicken breasts and onion and add enough water to cover. Cover the pan and poach over medium-low heat until the chicken is white throughout, about 20 minutes.

3. In the meantime, in a large frying pan, heat the olive oil over medium heat. Add the mushrooms and cook until tender, about 5 minutes.

4. Place the spinach in an 8-inch square baking dish. Sprinkle with the nutmeg, salt, and pepper.

5. Arrange the chicken in a single layer over the spinach. Top with the mushrooms.

6. Sprinkle evenly with the cheese and broil for 1 to 2 minutes, until the cheese is melted.

## Chicken Larb

*Serves 4, 2 filled leaves per serving*

This is a spicy dish from the northern region of Thailand. If you want to make it extra-spicy, use some Sriracha sauce to heat it up.

> 1 pound ground chicken (white meat)
> 2 tablespoons red curry paste
> ½ teaspoon sea salt
> 1 tablespoon canola oil
> ⅓ cup chopped English (seedless) cucumber
> ¼ cup chopped shallots
> 3 tablespoons chopped fresh cilantro
> 2 tablespoons fresh lime juice
> 8 cabbage or iceberg lettuce leaves
> Sriracha sauce (optional)

1. Combine the chicken, curry paste, and salt in a bowl.

2. Heat a large skillet over medium-high heat. Add the oil and swirl to coat.

3. Add the chicken and cook, stirring and breaking it up with a wooden spoon, until cooked through, about 6 minutes.
4. Remove the pan from the heat and stir in the cucumber, shallots, cilantro, and lime juice.
5. Divide the chicken mixture evenly among the cabbage leaves.
6. Serve with Sriracha sauce, if desired.

## Vinegar Chicken

*Serves 4*

2 tablespoons extra-virgin olive oil
1 (3-pound) chicken, cut up into serving pieces
4 garlic cloves, unpeeled
¼ teaspoon sea salt
Freshly ground black pepper
½ cup tarragon vinegar
1 (14.5-ounce) can chopped tomatoes
1 tablespoon chopped fresh parsley

1. In a large frying pan, heat the oil over medium heat.
2. Add the chicken and garlic. Cook, turning the chicken, until it is lightly browned, about 5 minutes per side. Season the chicken with the salt and pepper to taste.
3. Add the vinegar and bring to a boil. Then add the tomatoes and parsley.
4. Cover, reduce the heat to a simmer and cook until the chicken is tender, about 20 minutes.
5. Transfer the chicken to a serving platter and cover it loosely with aluminum foil to keep it warm.
6. Remove the garlic cloves, peel them under cold water, mash them, and return them to the sauce.
7. Pour the sauce over the chicken and serve.

## Pepper Chicken Casserole

*Serves 4*

This casserole is comfort food at its best. It's delicious warmed up the next day.

> 2 tablespoons extra-virgin olive oil
> 1¼ pounds boneless, skinless chicken breasts, cut into
>    1-inch cubes
> 2 medium red bell peppers, sliced
> 2 medium green bell peppers, sliced
> 2 cups sliced mushrooms
> 2 cups chopped onions
> ½ teaspoon dried oregano
> ½ teaspoon red pepper flakes
> ½ cup dry white wine
> 1 cup hot 2% milk

1.  Preheat the oven to 350°F.
2.  In a 2-quart flameproof casserole dish, heat the oil over medium-low heat.
3.  Add the chicken, bell peppers, mushrooms, onions, oregano, and red pepper flakes and cook until the chicken is opaque and the onions are tender, 5 to 8 minutes.
4.  Add the wine and cook for 5 minutes.
5.  Pour the hot milk over the chicken mixture and cover the casserole. Transfer to the oven and bake for 30 minutes.

## Tandoori Chicken

*Serves 4*

This Indian dish is colorful and has plenty of flavor. It's delicious served with a yogurt and cucumbers.

> 1½ cups 2% Greek yogurt
> 2 tablespoons grated onion

1 tablespoon grated peeled fresh ginger
1 tablespoon canola oil
½ teaspoon cayenne pepper
¼ teaspoon ground turmeric
3 garlic cloves, minced
4 boneless, skinless chicken breasts
½ teaspoon sea salt

1. Combine the yogurt, onion, ginger, oil, cayenne, turmeric, and garlic in a heavy-duty zip-top plastic bag.
2. Add the chicken to the bag and seal. Marinate in the refrigerator for 2 hours, turning occasionally.
3. Preheat the broiler to high. Place a small roasting pan in the oven.
4. Coat the preheated pan with cooking spray and place the chicken in the pan. Broil in the lower third of the oven for 15 minutes or until cooked through, turning after 7 minutes.

## Broiled Country Mustard Chicken

*Serves 4*

This effortless recipe is a keeper. When you are uninspired, this dish will come to the rescue with ingredients you have on hand. You can skip the scallions and garlic if you don't have them. You can also use granulated garlic, which should be in your pantry.

2 scallions, sliced
2 tablespoons coarse-grained mustard
2 tablespoons reduced-calorie mayonnaise
1 garlic clove, crushed through a press or minced
½ teaspoon dried basil
Freshly ground black pepper
4 boneless, skinless chicken breasts

1. Preheat the broiler.
2. Mix the scallions, mustard, mayonnaise, garlic, basil, and pepper to taste in a small bowl.
3. Place the chicken breasts on a broiling pan. Spread half the mustard mixture over the chicken.
4. Broil about 6 inches from the heat for 15 to 20 minutes, basting occasionally with the remaining mustard mixture.

## Turkey Piccata

*Serves 4, 2 cutlets per serving*

This recipe is great using chicken cutlets, too.

> 1½ pounds small turkey cutlets
> (about 8 cutlets at 3 ounces each)
> Sea salt and freshly ground black pepper
> 3 tablespoons extra-virgin olive oil
> ¼ cup chopped shallots
> 1 tablespoon sliced garlic
> ¾ cup dry white wine
> ½ cup low-sodium chicken stock
> 1 teaspoon almond flour
> 2 tablespoons fresh lemon juice
> 2 tablespoons capers, drained
> 2 tablespoons chopped fresh parsley

1. Season the turkey with salt and pepper.
2. Heat a skillet large enough to hold 4 cutlets over medium-high heat.
3. Add 1½ teaspoons of the oil to the pan and swirl to coat.
4. Put 4 of the cutlets in the pan and cook for about 2 minutes on each side, until cooked through. Remove the cutlets from the pan.
5. Repeat the procedure with 1½ teaspoons oil and the remaining cutlets.

6.  Add 1 tablespoon of extra-virgin olive oil to the pan, then add the shallots and garlic. Cook, stirring, for 2 minutes.
7.  Add the wine and increase the heat to high. Bring the wine to a boil and cook for 2 minutes, scraping the pan to loosen any browned bits stuck to the bottom.
8.  In a small bowl, whisk the chicken stock and almond flour together, add to the pan, and bring to a boil.
9.  Cook until the liquid has reduced by half, about 5 minutes.
10. Remove from the heat. Stir in the remaining 1 tablespoon olive oil, the lemon juice, and capers.
11. Pour the sauce over the cutlets and sprinkle with the parsley.

# Fish and Seafood

Fish used to be called "brain food." New research has found that weekly consumption of broiled or baked fish is associated with larger gray matter volume in areas of the brain responsible for memory and cognition. Aside from brainpower, fish are an excellent source of omega-3 fatty acids. Fish is a lean source of protein, which makes it an important component of the Change Your Biology Diet.

## Red Snapper Creole
*Serves 4*

A creole sauce can enhance so much food—from eggs to chicken, from fish and seafood to vegetables.

> 1 tablespoon extra-virgin olive oil
> ¼ cup chopped onion
> ¼ cup chopped green bell pepper
> 1 garlic clove, minced
> 1 (14.5-ounce) can whole tomatoes, chopped, juices reserved
> 2 teaspoons reduced-sodium Worcestershire sauce

2 teaspoons red wine vinegar
½ teaspoon dried basil
¼ teaspoon sea salt
Freshly ground black pepper
Dash of hot sauce
4 (6-ounce) red snapper fillets

1. In a large nonstick skillet, heat the oil over medium-high heat.
2. Add the onion, bell pepper, and garlic. Cook, stirring, until tender.
3. Add the tomatoes with their juices, Worcestershire, vinegar, basil, salt, black pepper, and hot sauce and bring to a boil.
4. Add the fillets. Spoon the tomato mixture over the fish. Reduce the heat, cover, and simmer until the fish flakes easily with a fork, about 12 minutes.

## Salmon with Red Pesto

*Serves 4*

The sauce from this quick recipe can be used with fish or chicken. It's a delicious variation on the pesto theme.

¾ teaspoon sea salt
4 (6-ounce) salmon fillets
⅓ cup chopped bottled roasted red peppers, drained and rinsed
7 blanched almonds
1 garlic clove
1 tablespoon tomato paste
1 teaspoon extra-virgin olive oil

1. Sprinkle ½ teaspoon of the salt on the fillets.
2. Heat a grill pan over medium-high heat. Coat the pan with cooking spray, then put the fish in the pan and cook until the

fish flakes easily with a fork or has reached the desired level of doneness, about 4 minutes on each side.

3. As the fish cooks, in a blender or food processor, combine the remaining ¼ teaspoon salt, the peppers, almonds, garlic, tomato paste, and olive oil and process until smooth.

4. Spoon the pesto over the salmon.

## Broiled Tilapia with Tangy Sauce
*Serves 4*

This fresh-tasting sauce works well with other fish and seafood, too.

> 1 tablespoon extra-virgin olive oil
> 4 (6-ounce) tilapia fillets
> Sea salt and freshly ground black pepper
> ¼ cup 2% Greek yogurt
> ¼ cup fresh lemon juice
> 2 tablespoons chopped fresh chives or scallions
> 1 teaspoon Dijon mustard

1. Preheat the broiler. Spray a baking dish big enough to hold the fillets without overlapping with cooking spray.

2. Drizzle the olive oil on both sides of the fillets. Brush to coat well. Season with salt and pepper.

3. Put the fish in the baking dish and broil for 8 minutes or until the fish flakes easily with a fork. Cover and set aside.

4. Combine the yogurt, lemon juice, chives, and mustard in a small bowl. Whisk to combine.

5. Arrange the fillets on a serving dish and spoon some sauce over each fillet.

# Seared Scallops with Cherry Tomatoes and Fennel
*Serves 4*

Fennel has a distinctive licorice flavor, which complements the sweet scallops. The tomatoes add color and texture.

3 tablespoons extra-virgin olive oil
16 sea scallops (about 1½ pounds)
½ teaspoon sea salt, plus more for the scallops
½ teaspoon freshly ground black pepper, plus more for the scallops
1 fennel bulb, thinly sliced, fronds chopped and reserved
1 small onion, thinly sliced
1 pint grape tomatoes
1 (8-ounce) bottle clam juice
½ cup dry white wine

1. In a large skillet, heat the oil over medium-high heat. Season the scallops with salt and pepper and cook on one side until just browned, 2 to 3 minutes. Transfer to a plate.
2. Add the sliced fennel, onion, salt, and pepper to the skillet. Stir occasionally and cook until the vegetables are just tender, 5 to 6 minutes.
3. Add the tomatoes, clam juice, and wine and cook until the liquid begins to thicken, 6 to 8 minutes.
4. Add the scallops, browned-side up, and cook until cooked through, 2 to 3 minutes more.
5. Sprinkle the scallops, vegetables, and liquid with 2 tablespoons of the reserved fennel fronds and serve.

# Sautéed Bass with Shiitake Mushroom Sauce
*Serves 4*

You can use this sauce on other fish, chicken, or beef. It works well with snapper and rainbow trout.

2 teaspoons canola oil
4 (6-ounce) skinless bass fillets
⅛ teaspoon sea salt
⅛ teaspoon freshly ground black pepper
2 cups sliced shiitake mushroom caps
1 teaspoon dark sesame oil
2 teaspoons ground ginger
1 teaspoon minced garlic
1 cup chopped scallions
¼ cup water
¼ cup low-sodium soy sauce
1 tablespoon fresh lemon juice

1. In a large nonstick skillet, heat the canola oil over medium-high heat.
2. Season the fish with the salt and pepper. Add the fish to the skillet and cook until the fish flakes easily with a fork, about 2½ minutes on each side. Remove the fish from the pan and cover it with aluminum foil to keep warm.
3. Add the mushrooms and sesame oil to the pan and cook, stirring, for 2 minutes.
4. Add the ginger and garlic and cook, stirring, for 1 minute.
5. Add the scallions, water, soy sauce, and lemon juice and cook, stirring, for 2 minutes.
6. Spoon the mushroom sauce over the fish.

## Parchment-Baked Halibut
*Serves 4*

This recipe will work with any white fish, such as cod, snapper, or sole. Cooking fish in parchment results in perfect texture and sweetness. (You can use heavy-duty foil instead, but it does not replicate cooking in parchment.)

4 (6-ounce) halibut fillets
4 tablespoons prepared pesto

1 cup shredded carrots (2 medium)
1 cup shredded zucchini (1 small)
¾ teaspoon sea salt
½ teaspoon freshly ground black pepper
4 teaspoons extra-virgin olive oil
4 teaspoons dry white wine

1. Preheat the oven to 450°F. Cut four 12 x 18-inch sheets of parchment paper or heavy-duty aluminum foil and coat the sheets with cooking spray, leaving a 2-inch border unsprayed.
2. Place the fillets on the lower side of the parchment paper, not touching the unsprayed border.
3. Spread 1 tablespoon of the pesto over each fillet and top each with ¼ cup of the carrots and ¼ cup of the zucchini. Season with the salt and pepper.
4. Drizzle 1 teaspoon of the oil and 1 teaspoon of the wine on each fillet. Fold the parchment paper and seal the edges with narrow folds.
5. Place the packets on rimmed baking sheets and bake for 15 minutes, or until the packets are puffy and lightly browned.
6. Serve the fish in the packets, piercing each so that steam can escape, or transfer the fillets to plates and top with the vegetables and juices.

## Broiled Flounder with Ginger-Lime Sauce

*Serves 4*

This high-flavor sauce works on fish, shrimp, scallops, and chicken. It's a treat for your taste buds.

1½ tablespoons extra-virgin olive oil
1 tablespoon chopped fresh cilantro
1 teaspoon minced seeded jalapeño pepper
½ teaspoon lime zest
¼ teaspoon ground ginger

¾ teaspoon sea salt
4 (6-ounce) flounder or other firm white-fleshed fish fillets
¼ teaspoon freshly ground black pepper
Lime wedges, for serving

1.  Combine the oil, cilantro, jalapeño, lime zest, and ginger in a bowl with ¼ teaspoon of the salt. Cover and chill.
2.  Heat a large nonstick skillet over medium-high heat. Coat the pan with cooking spray.
3.  Sprinkle both sides of the fish with the remaining ½ teaspoon salt and the pepper.
4.  Add the fish to the pan and cook until the fish flakes easily with a fork, about 3 minutes on each side.
5.  Transfer the fillets to plates or a serving platter and top each with 1½ teaspoons of the sauce. Serve with lime wedges.

# Beef

Most of my patients grill a steak or a burger when they eat beef. I am including a recipe for meat loaf, because the leftovers are so good.

## Blue Plate Special Meat Loaf
*Serves 8*

When you feel the need for comfort food, there is nothing quite like meat loaf. And what is better than meat loaf leftovers? Low-carb meat loaf leftovers. You can make individual meat loaves in a muffin tin and wrap some to freeze.

1 (8-ounce) can tomato sauce
1 (6-ounce) can tomato paste
¼ cup sugar substitute or low-calorie brown sugar
2 teaspoons distilled white vinegar
2 pounds 90% lean ground beef or turkey, or a combination
2 large eggs

½ cup grated Parmesan cheese

¼ cup diced red onion

¼ cup diced red bell pepper

2 tablespoons chopped fresh parsley (optional)

2 garlic cloves, minced

½ teaspoon dried basil

½ teaspoon dried oregano

Sea salt and freshly ground black pepper

1. Preheat the oven to 375°F.
2. In a small bowl, mix together the tomato sauce, tomato paste, sugar substitute, and vinegar. Add some water to make the mixture the consistency of ketchup.
3. In a medium bowl, mix together the meat, eggs, cheese, onion, bell pepper, parsley, garlic, basil, oregano, and salt and pepper to taste.
4. Pour half the tomato sauce into the meat mixture and mix with your hands.
5. Pack the meat into a loaf pan and even the top, or make individual loaves in muffin tins. Cover the top of the meat loaf with the remaining tomato sauce.
6. Bake for 45 to 50 minutes and let rest for 2 to 5 minutes before slicing.

# Sides

You can eat unlimited vegetables and salads. We haven't focused on side dishes, but wanted to provide you with some recipes that will expand your range.

## Roasted Vegetables

Crunchy roasted vegetables are a delicious side dish and snack. Brussels sprouts, broccoli, carrots, parsnips, eggplant, cauliflower, green beans, halved cherry tomatoes or tiny grape or plum tomatoes, onions, and butternut squash are delicious cooked this way. If you roast kale, you have kale chips, a nutritious alternative to potato chips. You can mix the vegetables for a colorful snack. You can combine roast vegetables with quinoa for a balanced meal when you have added grains to your diet. Experiment with seasoning when you roast. I like to use cumin on carrots or basil and garlic with the tomatoes. Always make extra roast vegetables. They could well become your favorite snack.

1. Preheat the oven to 350°F. Line a baking sheet with parchment paper to save on clean-up time.
2. Cut the vegetables into bite-size pieces or florets.
3. Put the vegetables in a plastic bag with a little extra-virgin olive oil—do not use too much oil. Shake to coat.
4. Spread the vegetables in a single layer on the lined baking sheet. Season with sea salt.
5. Bake for 25 to 45 minutes, depending on the size of the pieces, the tenderness of the vegetables, and how crisp you want them to be. Smaller pieces and tender veggies, like zucchini, cook quickly.

## Can't Believe It's Not Mashed Potatoes
*Serves 4*

If you need a potato fix, try this delicious cauliflower substitute. The texture is convincing, and the flavor is even better. Since everything goes into a food processor or blender, you can chop the cauliflower, including the top of the stems, and garlic coarsely. If you would like, you can add rosemary and/or thyme to the mash.

1 medium head cauliflower, cut into florets with the top of
    the stems

2 garlic cloves, sliced
1 tablespoon low-fat cream cheese, at room temperature
¼ cup grated Parmesan cheese
½ teaspoon sea salt
Freshly ground black pepper
Chopped fresh chives, for garnish

1. In a large pot fitted with a steamer basket, steam the cauliflower and garlic over simmering water until tender, 5 to 7 minutes.
2. In a blender or food processor, combine the cauliflower and garlic with the rest of the ingredients except chives and puree until close to smooth.
3. Garnish with fresh chives.

## Vegetable Quinoa
*Serves 6*

When you start to eat grains again, you should add quinoa to your diet. Quinoa is a nutritious grain that has a lot of protein. It's also a satisfying substitute for rice and pasta. Keep extra in your freezer and refrigerator. Try this basic recipe, and then create your own delicious combinations of your favorite vegetables. Be creative—you can use any kind of raw, sautéed, or roasted vegetables. Greens are especially delicious.

2 tablespoons extra-virgin olive oil
1 medium red onion, chopped
4 celery stalks, chopped
2 carrots, chopped
1 cup uncooked quinoa
2 cups water or low-sodium vegetable broth
4 garlic cloves
Sea salt and freshly ground black pepper
Fresh parsley or cilantro, for garnish

1.  Leave the vegetables raw, or for less crunch, in a medium saucepan, heat 1 tablespoon of the olive oil over medium-low heat, add the vegetables, and cook, stirring, until tender, about
    5 minutes.
2.  Rinse the uncooked quinoa in a fine-mesh strainer. Put the quinoa in a pot along with the water.
3.  Add the garlic cloves, remaining olive oil, and salt and pepper to taste and bring the liquid to a boil.
4.  Reduce the heat to low and simmer until all liquid has been absorbed by the quinoa, about 15 minutes.
5.  Mix in the vegetables.
6.  Garnish with parsley or cilantro.

## Hot Lentil Salad

*Serves 4, 1 cup per serving*

This is a delicious dish that you can eat cold, too. Lentils are nutritious and easy to make. You do not have to soak them overnight, and they cook quickly. Any amount of lentils can be cooked as described below. Just maintain the 2:1 ratio of water to lentils. Season them with olive oil, lemon juice, vinegar, and fresh herbs, or eat them on their own. Lentils can also be added to soups, salads, or other recipes.

1 cup brown or green lentils
2 cups water
1 bay leaf
¼ teaspoon sea salt, plus more as needed
¼ cup extra-virgin olive oil
2 zucchini, diced
4 celery stalks, sliced
1 onion, diced
¾ cup green beans, cut into short lengths
2 garlic cloves, crushed

½ red bell pepper, diced
½ yellow bell pepper, diced
1 tablespoon balsamic vinegar
1 teaspoon Dijon mustard
Freshly ground black pepper

1. Measure the lentils into a strainer or colander. Remove them any shriveled lentils, debris, or rocks. Thoroughly rinse the lentils under running water.
2. Transfer the rinsed lentils to a saucepan and pour in the water. Add the bay leaf.
3. Bring the water to a rapid simmer over medium-high heat, then reduce the heat to maintain a gentle simmer. You should only see a few small bubbles and some slight movement in the lentils. Cook, uncovered, for 20 to 30 minutes. Add water as needed to make sure the lentils are just barely covered. The lentils are done as soon as they are tender and no longer crunchy. Older lentils may take longer to cook and shed their outer skins as they cook. When done, drain the lentils and remove the bay leaf. Return the lentils to the pan and stir in the salt.
4. While the lentils are cooking, in a saucepan, heat the oil over medium heat. Add the zucchini, celery, onion, green beans, and garlic and cook for 5 minutes.
5. Add the bell peppers to the pan and cook for a minute more.
6. Stir in the vinegar and mustard.
7. Pour the warm vegetable mixture over the cooked lentils and toss. Season with salt and pepper.

# Baked Zucchini

*Serves 4*

This simple dish looks as good as it tastes. The thinly sliced zucchini cooks quickly and can trick you into thinking you are eating carbs.

2 medium zucchini, thinly sliced lengthwise
Sea salt
2 teaspoons extra-virgin olive oil
2 tablespoons Parmesan cheese

1. Preheat the oven to 400°F.
2. Lay the zucchini slices on a rimmed baking sheet in a single layer without overlapping.
3. Season with salt and drizzle the olive oil over the top. Sprinkle evenly with the Parmesan cheese.
4. Bake until the cheese starts to brown, about 5 minutes.

•  •  •

If you want to lose weight and keep it off, you have to do more than change your eating habits. To keep your metabolism revved up and fight your body's natural drive to regain the pounds you have lost, you have to become more physically active. The next chapter will show you that you don't have to dread exercise. Simply standing more can make a difference, and high-intensity resistance training only requires a twenty-minute commitment a week to build lean muscle mass. Read on.

# CHAPTER 10

# Stand Up and Start Moving

As you revise your diet, you have to build more movement into your life. Being physically active is an important component of the Change Your Biology program. Your diet alone will not get you where you want to be. You need to move more to fight weight loss resistance and to break through plateaus. You know that when you lose weight, your appetite-suppressing hormones fall dramatically, your hunger hormones rise, and your metabolism slows down. To keep burning fat, you need to expend more energy and create lean muscle mass.

The biggest complaint I hear from my patients is that they just don't have time to exercise. The fact is that improving your health and the shape of your body requires less exercise than you might think. Just as one size doesn't fit all with diets, how you move and build muscle depends on where you start. You don't have to train like a triathlete or work out two hours a day to see and feel positive change. Moving more in your everyday life and doing high-intensity strength training for less than ten minutes twice a week is enough to make a difference. If you are totally sedentary, you might start by just standing more during the day. If you are mostly sedentary, you can gradually add physical activity to your life. In time, you will be ready to do ten minutes of the Intro to High Intensity resistance training workout that follows twice a week. If you are active and work out regularly, you will find that increasing the intensity and decreasing the length of your workout can lead to great results and more free time. Working your muscles to exhaustion is the most effective way to build lean muscle, which will make your body a calorie-burning machine.

I do make a distinction between movement and exercise. You need both to raise your fitness level and to reverse the complications of weight gain. Movement can range from sitting for fewer hours a day all the way to doing yoga, hiking, taking a bike ride outside, or enjoying a Zumba class. One way to look at it is to think of movement as recreation—something you do for fun that restores and refreshes you. Everyone can use more of that.

To reduce body fat, burn calories more efficiently, and increase lean muscle mass, strength training is the answer. Later in the chapter, you will find three levels of workouts—Intro to High Intensity, High-Intensity Progress, and High-Intensity Peak—designed by Adam Zickerman, one of the pioneers of slow-movement, high-intensity resistance training. Each workout consists of eight exercises that can be done in less than ten minutes. You will increase the intensity of your workout as you get stronger. To start, you have to realize what being inactive does to you. It all begins with sitting for too many hours a day.

# The Sitting Disease

Researchers and medical experts refer to the negative consequences of long periods of physical inactivity as the "sitting disease." Sitting for long periods of time has been linked to obesity, metabolic syndrome, and a number of other health concerns. Too much chair time appears to increase the risk of death from cardiovascular disease and cancer. Several studies have produced some sobering statistics:

- One recent study compared a group of adults who spent less than two hours a day in front of the television, computer, or tablet with another group who watched more than four hours a day. Those who logged more hours in front of a screen in their leisure time had an almost 50 percent increased risk of death from any cause and about a 125 percent increased risk of cardiovascular disease.

- The *New York Times* reported on an Australian study that found that every hour of television watched after the age of twenty-five reduced the viewer's life expectancy by 21.8 minutes. In comparison, smoking a cigarette reduces life expectancy by 11 minutes. Other media ran with the tagline: "Sitting is more dangerous to your health than smoking."

- In the same Australian study, those who sat the most had a 112 percent increase in their risk of developing diabetes, a 147 percent risk for cardiovascular disease, and a 49 percent risk of dying prematurely.

- The American Cancer Society looked at the health of 123,000 Americans between 1991 and 2006. Men who spent six hours or more a day of their leisure time sitting had a death rate 20 percent higher than men who sat for three hours or less. Women who sat for more than six hours a day in their leisure time had a death rate about 40 percent higher than those who were more active.

If you think that watching your diet and going to the gym a few times a week will make up for your time being sedentary, your assumption has been proven incorrect. Spending a few hours a week doing moderate or vigorous activity does not appear to offset the risk of too much sedentary time. Even if you exercise thirty minutes a day, you should consider how active you are for the other twenty-three hours and thirty minutes of your day.

Today, most people spend the majority of the day sitting at their desks, at conference room tables, in restaurants, in their cars, on buses, or on trains while commuting, and then sit in front of a computer or television when they get home. People even shop with a click of a mouse, never leaving their chairs. Americans adults spend 55 to 70 percent of their time sitting or lying on a couch, ranging from 7.7 to 15 hours of waking time. When you count hours spent sleeping, say, seven, being sedentary can add up to twenty-two hours. It is clear that we have to get out of those chairs and move more.

When you sit, electrical activity in your muscles drops. When muscles do not contract, especially the large and powerful muscles of the legs and buttocks, there are metabolic consequences. The muscles require less fuel, and blood sugar accumulates in the bloodstream, which contributes to diabetes risk. One study of healthy, thin young men showed a 40 percent drop in the effectiveness of insulin after twenty-four hours of being sedentary. The enzymes that break down triglycerides and lipids and help clean harmful fat out of the bloodstream fall, resulting in lower good cholesterol levels. The rate at which you burn calories plummets to a calorie a minute, a third of what your body would burn if you got up and walked.

Sitting also affects your genes and can cause your cells to die prematurely. Telomeres are the protective caps at the end of DNA strands. They are like the tips of shoelaces. When you lose that plastic tip, your shoelaces start to fray. In the same way, telomeres prevent DNA strands from unraveling and dying.

A Swedish study of sedentary, overweight, sixty-eight-year-old men and women found that reduced sitting time was associated with lengthening the telomeres. Their cells appeared to be growing physiologically younger. There was a negative correlation between exercise and telomere length. Those who exercised the most during the six-month study tended to have some shortening of their telomeres, compared to those who exercised less but stood up more.

It turns out that just standing more is good for you. This idea originated in the 1950s when a study was done in England that compared bus conductors, who stand collecting tickets, to bus drivers, who sit. The study showed that the bus conductors had about half the risk of developing heart disease as the bus drivers. Recent studies have shown that when you stand, you burn more calories. Heart rates were much higher in the study's standing group, which translates to burning more calories a minute. Depending on your size, standing may help you burn an additional twenty to fifty calories an hour.

In a recent study, sixteen non-gym-goers were overfed by 1,000 calories a day and went about their normal lives. Some of the volunteers stored almost every single extra calorie as fat, while others did not gain an ounce. The people who spent most of the day seated gained weight, and those who moved around stayed slim. The reason is what is called NEAT, or non-exercise activity thermogenesis, which is the energy expended for everything you do that is not sleeping, eating, or exercise—in other words, the many minor movements you make each day. The researchers found that the people who did not gain weight were unconsciously moving around more. It was as if their bodies had a switch that was activated when they overate. The bodies of the non-gainers automatically made the adjustment to deal with excess calories by moving more. Their bodies responded by making more small movements than they had before the overfeeding began, like taking the stairs or fidgeting. The subjects who gained weight sat an average of two more hours a day than those who did not.

## Inactivity Changes Your Brain and Your Microbiome

While research has shown that regular exercise is good for your gray matter, stimulating the brain to form new connections, run more efficiently, and produce new neurons, an animal study done a year ago found that inactivity can also change brain structure. The neurons in the brains of rats that had been inactive for three months during the study were significantly different from a group that had been active over the same three-month period. The researchers were looking at a part of the brain that helps to oversee the sympathetic nervous system, which controls many of the body's constant needs, including heart rate, breathing, and blood pressure. They found that in the sedentary rats, the neurons in this part of the brain had changed shape and sprouted more branches. These branches made the neurons easily overstimulated. The changed neurons sent confusing messages to the nervous system, which ultimately caused blood pressure to rise and contributed to cardiovascular disease. Though this has not yet been studied in humans, this section of the brain in rats is similar to the area in our brains that controls the same systems. Just as eating sugary foods damages your brain, there is a good chance that inactivity does as well.

One intriguing study, done in Ireland, found that being physically active may encourage beneficial germs to thrive in the gut, influencing weight and overall health by changing the composition of the microbiome, and that inactivity could do the reverse. The researchers chose forty professional rugby players, who were exercising strenuously for several hours a day. They recruited two other groups of men who were not athletes. One group had a normal BMI and exercised occasionally. The third group consisted of men who had a BMI in the overweight or obese range and who were mostly sedentary. The rugby players had more diversity in their gut microbiome than the other groups. The rugby players' guts contained larger numbers of a bacterium that has been linked with a decreased risk for obesity and inflammation. The men in the other groups, especially those with the highest BMI, had low levels of this bacterium and high markers for inflammation in their bloodstream. This is a preliminary study that did not consider diet. The athletes had eaten far more calories than the other men, and their diet was very high in protein. As you know, what you eat affects the composition of the microbiome in your gut. The researchers are now studying men and women. I thought this study was worth mentioning, because it is innovative. It is the beginning of an examination of the effect of physical activity or lack of it on the community of microbes that live in your body.

I have extensively covered these new findings about the connection of inactivity to your health because I want you to understand how important it is to move. Even if you have severe obesity, you can begin your commitment to exercise by simply standing more. There are so many ways you can get up and add movement to your life. You don't have to buy a "treadmill desk" or a "stand-up desk," the hot new office furnishings, to see and feel results. You do not have to exhaust yourself with a rigorous and time-consuming workout that you will end up abandoning, as you probably have in the past if you are like many of my patients. You do not have to waste money on a gym membership and feel guilty for never going. You just have to take it slow and steady, beginning with building routine movement into your life. It's about breaking couch potato habits.

# 40 Ways to Get Active

There are so many easy things you can do that will get you on your feet and moving. This doesn't have to be torture. Making slight adjustments in your daily routine will get you going. After you have upped your movement, you will likely find yourself feeling so much better that you will want to incorporate even more movement into your daily life. The key is to find activities that you enjoy and look forward to doing. Being active should be a pleasurable part of your life. Here are some simple things you can do to move more:

1.  Take a fifteen-minute walk after each meal. One study showed that when subjects sat down after a meal, their blood sugar skyrocketed and stayed high for about two hours. A leisurely post-meal stroll reduced blood sugar levels by half.

2.  No matter what you are doing, get up every twenty minutes and walk twenty feet or stand for two minutes.

3.  Set the timer on your phone to go off every 20 minutes to remind you get up.

4.  Get an anti-sitting app such as Time Out or Break Reminder that lets you know when it's time to get up. In the past, people used to take smoking and coffee breaks. Skip the nicotine and caffeine, but do get up and get some fresh air.

5.  Find a movement buddy who has the same goal as you. It will make it more fun.

6.  Stand for all or part of your commute if you take a bus, train, or subway.

7.  Get off public transportation a stop earlier and walk to your destination.

8.  Park your car farther away in a parking lot or a block or two away from where you are going.

9.  Take the stairs—or at least a few flights—and skip the elevator or escalator.

10. Stand and pace when you talk on the phone.

11. If you can't leave your chair, fidget. Little movements count, though they may be distracting or send the wrong message in a meeting.

12. Get up to get water every odd or even hour—whether it's walking to the water cooler or going to the kitchen for bottled, filtered, or tap water. You will not only be moving, but you will also be well hydrated.

13. If you are going out for lunch or picking up food to eat at your desk, chose a place that is a nice walk from your office or home.

14. Eat lunch at a standing counter now and then.

15. Put away your remote controls. Change channels and volume manually.

16. Don't carry your cell phone around with you in your house or apartment. Leave it in a designated place so that you have to get up to answer it when it rings.

17. While you're at it, if you have a landline, leave the receiver in the charging station.

18. Use a stationary chair at your desk so you have to get up rather than just roll to get things you need.

19. Stretch at your desk regularly during the day.

20. Rather than sending an e-mail, go to your colleague's office to discuss what's on your mind.

21. Take meetings outside your office. Either go to someone else's office or a conference room or invite a coworker to take a stroll to discuss the matter at hand.

22. Don't make things too convenient at the office. Place office supplies and files away from your desk so that you have to get out of your chair to get what you need.

23. Clear off your desk at the end of the day. Stand as you go through papers and put them away.

24. Stand when you are having a drink at a bar.

25. Rather than sit in a coffee shop, meet a friend for a walk and carry your coffee with you.

26. Walk a dog. If you don't have one, volunteer at an animal shelter or borrow a friend's or neighbor's pet.

27. Go for a bike ride.

28. Listen to audiobooks or podcasts while you are doing chores or errands rather than curling up in a chair to read.

29. Spend time with children. That will keep you active. If you don't have children of your own, babysit for a relative or friend or volunteer to work with kids.

30. Explore local parks on foot.

31. Don't have food delivered. Go pick it up instead.

32. Take up gardening.

33. Play music and dance while you do housework.

34. When you are watching TV, get up during commercials and stretch, do a chore, or work out your arms with dumbbells rather than going to the refrigerator.

35. Learn a new sport.

36. Wear a pedometer or an activity tracker. They are great motivators to move more.

37. If you are a gamer, try an active Wii game instead of sitting to play.

38. Check out the yoga channels on YouTube and find a yoga teacher who works for you.

39. Find a cable exercise channel. It's like having a personal trainer in your own home.

40. Join a club or team organized around an activity, such as rowing, hiking, biking, ballroom dancing, or bird-watching, so that you make new friends who are active.

You should feel better once you start moving more. And as you lose weight, you should find it easier to move. Being physically active can tap into reserves of energy you did not know you had. Moving more will improve your mood, increase your optimism, and generally improve the quality of your life. It's so easy to become lethargic. You are surrounded by energy-saving devices and ways to accomplish things. What are you saving that energy for? The energy you save is being converted to fat. Your goal is to become an energy-burning furnace. The best way to do that is to build lean muscle mass.

## Cut the Time, Increase the Intensity

I have made a distinction between movement and exercise, because exercise supports change, but not the way exercise used to be defined. Jogging on a treadmill at a steady, moderate pace for thirty minutes or more—or "doing cardio"—does not burn much fat. You do not have to spend hours a week on a stationary bike, elliptical machine, or treadmill. High-intensity interval training has been shown to burn much more fat in less time than steady-state cardio workouts. High-intensity interval training involves bursts of high-intensity exercise, for example, running at 90 percent of your maximum heart rate, followed by a low-intensity interval, such as walking at a moderate pace. The reason interval training works so well is that a greater calorie burn, due to increased post-exercise oxygen consumption, is maintained after the workout is over. When you exercise this way, you increase your resting metabolism, which means you burn more calories and body fat while doing nothing.

The *New York Times* reported that researchers at the University of Copenhagen in Denmark have developed a new approach to high-intensity interval training that makes it less challenging. They found that even though high-intensity training was an effective way to improve health, many people did not like to push themselves and stopped the training. They call their low-tech routine 10-20-30 training. This is how it works:

- Run, ride a bike, or work out on an elliptical or rowing machine gently for 30 seconds.

- Speed up to a moderate pace for 20 seconds.

- Sprint as hard as you can for 10 seconds.

- Repeat 4 times.

- Rest for 2 minutes by walking slowly or standing.

- Repeat 5 intervals.

The entire session lasts 12 minutes. You can add another set of 5 intervals when you feel ready. This workout should not be done on consecutive days.

Physical activity of any kind lowers and regulates blood sugar levels, because when muscles contract, they draw sugar from the bloodstream for fuel. In one study of people with insulin resistance, a group who walked at a moderate pace for thirty minutes before dinner lowered their post-meal blood sugar level, as would be expected. Another group did three quick sessions of interval training a day before meals. Their workout consisted of one minute of brisk walking followed by another minute of strolling, repeated six times—twelve

Ashley is a forty-three-year-old publicist who works with celebrities. She has a five-year-old-son and two stepchildren. Handling it all with good grace drives her stress levels through the roof. She came to see me when her weight hit 222 pounds. Her BMI was 35.8.

When we discussed her lifestyle, she said her problem was not binge-ing. She ate out six to eight times a week because of work. Eating out that often can easily lead to weight gain. Not only are portion sizes large, but unless you special order, you have no idea what ingredients the cook is using to make the food taste good. Ashley always started the day with a high-carb breakfast. She would grab a muffin in the green room of TV shows when accompanying a celebrity or eat something from a local bak-ery at her desk. She agreed to try a low-carb, high-protein diet. I prescribed metformin to improve her insulin resistance. Her cravings disappeared. She worked out more. Ashley lost twenty pounds in six months.

With her weight down to 202 pounds, she continued with metformin and I added Topamax. While she was losing an additional ten pounds, she relied on support from my staff about her diet, checking in with them regu-larly. She found that she had a lot more energy after losing twenty pounds. She started to go to the gym four times a week and did some spinning. I added Wellbutrin to her other medications.

In four months, she weighed 173 pounds—an additional nineteen-pound loss. That put her total loss to thirty-nine pounds, a 17.6 percent loss of her total weight. She went to Paris for an event and was so in con-trol that she could have a bite of a baguette and stop there. Two months later, she was down to 166. She was breaking through plateaus as if they did not exist.

She kept up her exercise and eating and got down to 162 pounds. But then her weight started to go up gradually, two or three pounds every few months, until she was up to 168. She found herself craving carbs. Since the urge to eat was worst in the evenings, we changed the time she took her Topamax to before dinner. I increased her dose of Wellbutrin. Ashley's weight trended down again and she lost two pounds. She was glad she could fit into her dress for the Oscars.

Her weight started to rise again during the build-up to the Oscars, because of all the parties, late nights, complimentary food, and stress.

She was on her feet a lot at events, but was too tired to do high-intensity workouts. It drove home the point that anyone who has lost a lot of weight has to exercise. She needed to exercise to overcome weight loss resistance. She got up a half hour earlier each day and went for a twelve-minute interval training session at the hotel's gym. If the place she was staying didn't have a gym, she tied on her running shoes and did intervals outside.

When things quieted down after the Oscars and post-Oscar appearances, we added phentermine to her regimen for a short time. Her weight has stabilized at 170, and she keeps it there, because she hasn't stopped moving. She now takes Topamax, metformin, and Contrave to help to maintain a weight at which she is comfortable and a BMI of 27.4.

minutes three times a day. The researchers call this form of interval training "exercise snacks." The group who did the "snacks" lowered their blood sugar for twenty-four hours. This study suggests that interval exercise every other day is just as effective as continuous exercise every day for regulating blood sugar.

The key to high-intensity exercise is to exert yourself. When you are doing a high-intensity interval, your level of exertion should be a nine on a scale of ten. High-intensity exercise changes your muscles and body at the cellular level. Strenuous exertion activates a single protein that integrates signals from two different pathways to direct muscle growth.

In an animal study, researchers looked at how strenuous exercise affects the sympathetic nervous system. The sympathetic nervous system controls important automatic mechanisms like temperature adjustment. It sets off the fight-or-flight response as a reaction to danger or stress, and your body goes into high alert and mobilizes resources. In the stress response, the sympathetic nervous system stimulates the release of adrenaline and norepinephrine, which are biochemicals called catecholamines that make the heart race, increase alertness, and get oxygen and energy to the muscles to fuel escape or confrontation. The scientists wanted to study the relationship between the stress biochemical and CRTC2, a protein that is genetically activated during stress. When you exercise intensely, you set off the stress response and the CRTC2 protein is released.

They studied a group of mice that were genetically programmed to produce more CRTC2 than normal mice. These mice did a program of strenuous treadmill running. Their endurance soared by 103 percent after two weeks. The normal mice improved by 8.5 percent doing the same routine. The genetically modified animals developed larger muscles than the control group. Their muscle size increased by 15 percent. Their bodies grew more efficient at releasing fat from muscles to use as fuel. The protein was receiving signals from the catecholamines and passed those chemical messages to genes in muscle cells that set off processes that produced stronger muscles. This experiment shows how high intensity exercise helps to build muscles. **What this means for you is that if you do not get out of your comfort zone when you exercise, you will not trigger as strong a response and your workouts will not be as effective.**

## Turn White Fat to Brown

As you will remember, when you get cold, brown fat acts like a muscle and burns calories, taking fat from the rest of the body for fuel. New research is revealing the potential of brown fat for weight control and producing questions that have yet to be answered. Just three years ago, researchers thought brown fat was found only in rodents, which cannot shiver to generate heat to stay warm, and human infants, for the same reason. The assumption was that adults had no need for it. Scientists have since found a few ounces of brown fat in adults located along the spine, on the upper back, the side of the neck, and between the collarbone and the shoulder. They found stores of brown fat with scans of these areas when subjects were cold. Further scans revealed that brown fat burns ordinary fat. When brown fat cells use up their small stores of fat, they draw fat out of the rest of the body. This type of fat can fuel itself with triglycerides taken from the bloodstream known to increase the risk of developing metabolic syndrome. In addition, brown fat cells can draw sugar from the blood, which could help lower the risk for type 2 diabetes.

Another type of brown fat has been identified in mice. It is distributed in white fat. In mice, exercise can convert white fat to brown. During exercise, the muscle cells in mice release irisin, a hormone that stimulates white fat to behave like brown fat. In one study, researchers injected mice with a gene that tripled the levels of irisin in the blood of obese mice with very high glucose levels. The mice lost weight and gained control of their glucose levels in just ten days. Scientists speculate that some of the effects of human exercise, which has been found to make brown fat more active, might be explained by the presence of irisin in our blood.

This field of research is exploring new treatments for obesity based on brown fat. One of the goals is to learn how to keep stores of brown fat as large and active in adulthood as they are in infancy. Until breakthroughs in this field are made, you can activate your brown fat by being cold or with exercise.

## Work Those Muscles

High-intensity workouts can apply to resistance training as well as cardio. I have asked Adam Zickerman, an expert on high-intensity weight training, owner of InForm Fitness, and author of the *New York Times* best-seller *Power of 10*, to create three high-intensity workouts you can do at home with a minimum of equipment. Light dumbbells would be good to have, but you can use anything with weight that you can hold, like a quart or half-gallon jug of milk. He has designed three full-body programs to suit varying levels of fitness: Intro to High Intensity, High-Intensity Progress, and High-Intensity Peak. These routines have to be done super-slowly, because moving with control makes them safe and effective. I have asked Adam to introduce the workouts:

"After more than thirty years of pounding the pavement or running on a noisy treadmill, Americans are not fit, not in shape, and not lean. Endless aerobic sessions do not seem to be the answer. Most fitness experts agree that the key to fitness and weight loss is resistance training. Only resistance training builds lean muscle mass, which not only makes you look better but also burns more calories.

Three extra pounds of lean muscle burns about ten thousand extra calories a month just to sustain itself. **Having three extra pounds of muscle burns as many calories as running twenty-five miles a week without having to leave your couch.**

"My strength and conditioning program for *The Change Your Biology Diet* centers on slowing the pace of resistance training and fatiguing every muscle fiber twice a week. Each workout takes ten minutes or less. Even the world's busiest person can spare twenty minutes a week. The workouts I have designed can be done at home without any equipment but a wall, a chair, and 2.5- or 5-pound weights — a can of beans or a jug of detergent will do in a pinch. Most of the exercises use the weight of your own body as the resistance.

"The best way to build muscle is to slowly lift a moderately light weight, including parts of your body, until the muscle you are working is exhausted. Each time you move the weight, you lift ten seconds up and ten seconds down. One rep lasts 20 seconds. The continuous motion during the exercise keeps the tension of the weight in the muscle, not the joint. That way your muscles reach the point of fatigue efficiently and safely. Once the movement is complete, you do it again without resting, and then again, until you can no longer move your muscles. If you are doing a static exercise, hold a position until you can no longer. Your muscles will burn, you shake, and you are in 'muscle failure.' You do not have to count reps or sets with these routines. The slow movement works to build muscle without any harmful side effects or risks normally associated with high-intensity workouts — no wear-and-tear on joints, ligaments, or other connective tissue.

"**The most important aspect of the workout is intensity. Muscles have to be worked to the point of failure.** That means working a muscle group until you have no more force left to give. Not even an ounce, no matter how hard you push. I call it hitting the wall. You are fighting against the weight, unable to move another inch or hold a position a moment longer. This can be very uncomfortable. 'Go for the burn' applies here.

"Once you reach the point of failure, you cross this threshold and continue to push, counting to ten, even though you can't move the weight, repeat the movement, or can barely get your body off the floor. That final ten seconds, once you pass the point of failure, is the payoff. It's when change happens. If you push yourself to that level, you will collect the real prize. It is critical to understand the level of intensity required for results. It is easy to stop short. Most people work out at 80 percent. Working muscles until exhaustion, you have to keep doing reps until the muscles you are working cannot move.

"When you exercise to muscle exhaustion, you must allow the time for the muscles to rest so that your body can respond and start the muscle-building process. Rest and recovery is a significant part of the program. That is why you only need to do the workout twice a week. After each workout, you should rest your muscles for three or four days for proper muscle recovery. Overdoing these workouts is actually counterproductive. In the long term, these high-intensity resistance training workouts will allow you to maintain an exceptional level of strength and fitness for a lifetime.

"Remember that force causes injury. You impose force by using speed. If you slow down and lighten the weight, you get greater benefits. If the exercise requires you to repeat a motion, count slowly to ten up and then ten down. By lowering the speed, you are making the workout safer. Your muscles are doing all the work. You are not using momentum to help you to accelerate your reps, which translates as ultimate efficiency. The exercises in the workouts are biomechanically correct, designed to get the most from each exercise without stressing the joint. By tweaking familiar exercises with small changes in positions, I have shifted the axis of the movements to use force and resistance in the most efficient way to build muscle.

"My clients are surprised by how much their stamina increases. I keep a chart for each of my clients on which I record how long it takes them to reach muscle exhaustion on each exercise. You might want to consider using a stopwatch or timer to see how long you are able to do each exercise. It's a good way to measure your improvement. Remember to take it slow, and when you are ready to give up, don't. Just hold on another ten seconds. You can do it!

"If you have not done high-intensity training before, I advise you to start at the first level to get used to it. Your level of fitness determines how long it will take you to reach muscle exhaustion, so Level 1 will give anyone a good workout. The challenge is intensity."

# Level 1: Intro to High Intensity

This series of eight exercises is a full-body workout. Remember: **The key to making the exercises as effective as possible is to move slowly in a controlled way.**

Since you are working your muscles hard, you need to give them time to rest and relax. It is actually counterproductive to do this program more than twice a week. Try for one session on the weekend and one midweek. It should not take you more than ten minutes each time. If it does go over ten minutes, you are ready to move to the next level. You can keep doing this routine, but moving on will give you better results. Muscles have memory and your body gets used to a routine, so the exercises become less effective, unless you increase the intensity. That means you will have to exercise longer for the same result. It's smarter to move on to more challenging moves.

LEGS

## Exercise 1: Squats

Target: *buttocks and thighs*

1. Stand with your legs about hip-width apart. Extend your arms in front of you with your palms facing each other.

2. Bend your knees, hinge at your hips, and push your butt back as if you are about to sit

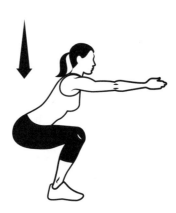

in a chair. Count to 10 on your way into position. Keep your back extended or straight. Make sure your knees are over your feet.

3. Press into the heels and come back up to a count of 10. Go slowly and use control.

4. Repeat until you cannot do another one, then try again and hold for 10 seconds.

For a greater challenge: Hold 2.5- or 5-pound weights. If you don't have weights, hold soup cans, laundry detergent jugs, or other weighted objects.

## Exercise 2: Calf Raise

Target: *lower leg*

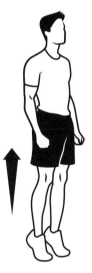

1. From a standing position, slowly rise up on your toes to a count of 10, keeping your knees straight and your heels off the floor.

2. Hold briefly, and then come back down to a count of 10.

3. Repeat slowly until your muscles are exhausted and you cannot do another one, then go halfway up and hold for 20 seconds.

### UPPER BODY

Push-ups are one of the most efficient upper body exercises out there. The problem is, most of us find push-ups difficult to perform. To overcome this, all you need is the right variation. The push-up comes in many forms—you will find increasingly challenging push-ups in the three workouts.

## Exercise 3: Wall Push-Up

Target: *front of shoulders, back of arms, chest, and upper back*

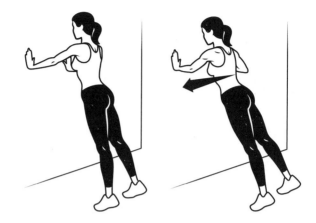

1. Stand facing a wall with your hands shoulder-width apart and your arms parallel to the floor. Your feet should be together, roughly 2 feet away from the wall.

2. Similar to a regular push-up, simply bend at the elbows and bring your chest toward the wall instead of the floor to a count of 10.

3. Push back to the starting position to a count of 10.

4. Repeat until your muscles are exhausted, then push away from the wall, stop halfway, and hold for 10 seconds.

For a greater challenge: Move your feet slightly farther away from the wall.

## Exercise 4: Seated Dumbbell Triceps Extension

Target: *triceps*

1. Sit on a flat bench or chair with a low back. Hold a 2.5- or 5-pound dumbbell securely with both hands, and raise it above your head with your arms extended. Make sure to keep a little bend in the elbows.

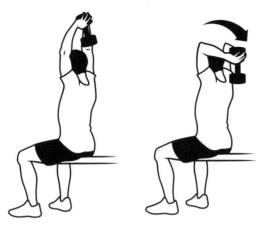

2. Slowly lower your arms behind your head to a count of 10. Keep your elbows in and all the tension in your triceps.

3. Slowly raise the dumbbell back up to the starting position to a count of 10 with your elbows held in.

4. Repeat until muscle exhaustion, then lower the weights halfway and hold for 10 seconds.

CORE

## Exercise 5: Back Extension

Target: *abs and back*

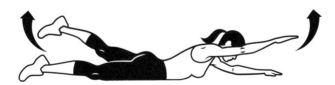

1. Lie on your stomach on a towel or mat with your arms stretched out in front of you.

2. Raise one hand and the opposite leg slightly off the floor to a count of 10 and pause briefly.

3.  Lower your hand and foot to a count of 10.

4.  Raise your other hand and opposite leg, pause, and lower.

5.  Alternate sides until you reach muscle exhaustion, then hold for 10 seconds on each side.

## Exercise 6: Knee Plank

Target: *abs, spine, and lower back*

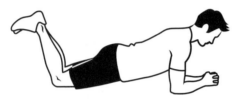

1.  Get down on your elbows and knees with your hands clasped. Create as much distance as you can between your elbows and knees by walking your knees back. Keep your back straight.

2.  Keep your abdominals held tight to support the lower back, and keep your head aligned with the spine by looking directly down at your clasped hands without dropping your head forward. Hold this position until you are no longer able to.

3.  Build up to at least 30 seconds before attempting a more challenging plank position.

## Exercise 7: Glute Bridge

Target: *hamstrings and butt*

1.  Lie on your back with your knees bent, your feet hip-width apart, and your arms at your side.

2.  Lift up your spine and hips. Keep your butt up. Only your head, feet, arms, and shoulders should be on the ground.

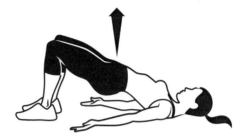

3.  Hold this position until exhaustion and then count to 10.

4.  Lower your spine gradually.

### ABS

## Exercise 8: Static Crunch

Target: *upper and lower abs*

1.  Lie on your back with your knees bent, feet flat, and arms at shoulder height, palms facing each other, reaching for the ceiling.

2.  Slowly roll up from the floor with your chin tucked. Just a slight lift is all that is necessary. Keep your arms reaching for the ceiling as if you are trying to pierce the ceiling with your fingertips.

3.  Hold the position until muscle exhaustion.

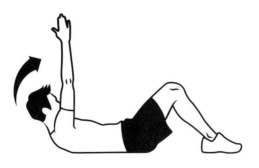

4. Then lower your spine a bit and hold for 10 seconds.

5. Lower yourself to resting position.

# Level 2: High-Intensity Progress

It's time to challenge your muscles with a new set of moves and variations on exercises from Level 1. Increase your intensity to build muscle mass.

### LEGS

## Exercise 1: Wall Sit

Target: *thighs and butt*

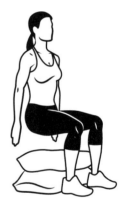

1. Place some pillows or a low backless stool between you and a wall.

2. Slowly slide your back down the wall until your thighs are parallel to the ground. Make sure your knees are directly above your ankles and keep your back straight.

3. Hold the position. Go for 60 seconds or however long it takes to turn your legs to jelly.

4. Rise up slowly to a count of 10.

## Exercise 2: Elevated Calf Raise

Do not try to balance on your own while doing this exercise. Make sure you are holding on to the back of a chair or a stair railing while you do these calf raises.

Target: *lower leg*

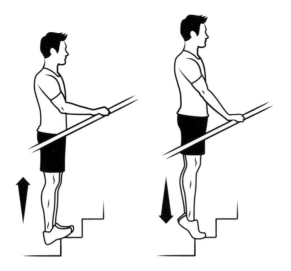

1.  Stand on something elevated such as a thick book, a sturdy stool, or a stair while holding on to the back of a chair or a railing. The elevation will allow you to achieve a wider range of motion when you drop your heels.

2.  Slowly rise up on your toes to a count of 10, keeping your knees straight and your heels off the floor.

3.  Hold briefly, and then drop your heels below your standing surface to a count of 10. Do not push it— a drop of an inch or two is fine.

4.  Rise up on your toes and repeat slowly until your muscles are exhausted and you cannot do another one, then go halfway up and hold for 20 seconds.

**UPPER BODY**

## Exercise 3: Push-Up from the Knees

This push-up is performed in the traditional method, except your knees act as the pivot point instead of your toes.

Target: *upper body*

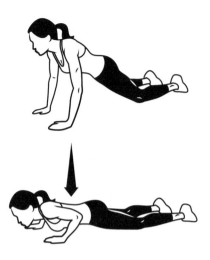

1. Get down on your knees and place your hands shoulder-width apart on the floor in front of you.

2. Slowly bend your arms at the elbow and lower your chest as close to the floor as you can to a count of 10. Tighten your abs and don't let your back sag. Hold your body in a straight line from your knees to the top of your head to keep your butt from pointing up in the air. Keep your head in a neutral position in line with the spine, eyes down.

3. Lift your body slowly by straightening your arms to a count of 10. Remember to keep your abs tight.

4. Repeat until muscle exhaustion, then raise yourself halfway and count to 10.

## ARMS

## Exercise 4: Seated Two-Handed Dumbbell Extension

Target: *triceps*

1. Sit on a flat bench, holding a 2.5- to 5-pound dumbbell securely in each hand.

2. Slowly raise the dumbbells above your head with your arms extended. Make sure to keep a little bend in your elbows while extending your arms.

3. Lower your arms down behind your head in a controlled way to a count of 10 while keeping your elbows in and all the tension on your triceps.

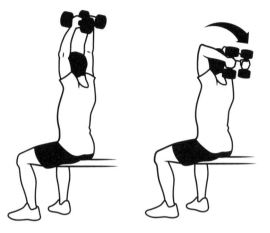

4. Slowly raise the dumbbell back to the starting position overhead to a count of 10 while keeping your elbows in throughout the movement.

5. Repeat this movement until muscle exhaustion.

CORE

## Exercise 5: Back Extension

Target: *abs and back*

1. Lie face down on the floor with your arms at your sides.

2. Keep your lower body and arms stationary and slowly raise your chest off the floor as you breathe out to a count of 10.

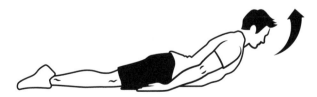

3. Pause for a moment and lower your chest slowly to the floor to a count of 10.

4. Repeat this movement until your muscles are exhausted. Then raise your chest up just a little and count to 10.

Another option is to keep the upper body stationary, and only raise the lower body off the ground.

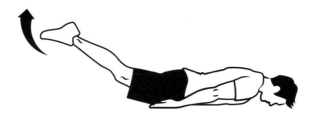

**ABS**

## Exercise 6: Full Plank

Target: *abs, spine, and lower back*

1. Lie face down with your forearms on the floor and hands clasped.

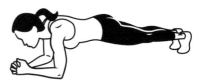

2. Rise up on your toes, keeping your back straight.

3. Tighten your core and hold the position as long as you can.

4. Lower yourself slowly to the floor.

## Exercise 7: Glute Bridge

Target: *hamstrings and butt*

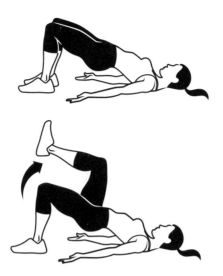

1. Lie on your back with your knees bent, feet hip-width apart, and arms at your sides.

2. Lift your spine and hips from the floor with only your head, feet, arms, and shoulders on the ground. Keep your spine straight.

3. Lift one leg upward to a count of 10 as you keep your core tight.

4. Slowly bring your leg down to a count of 10.

5. Then lift it back up.

6. Do this until muscle exhaustion. Lower your spine slowly back to the floor.

7. Lift your hips and spine again and repeat with the other leg.

## Exercise 8: Double Crunch

Target: *upper and lower abs*

1. Lie on your back with your knees bent, feet flat, and arms crossed at your chest.

2. While slowly rolling up from the floor with your chin tucked, lift your knees and feet off the ground with your knees bent at a 90 degree angle.

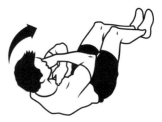

3. Hold the position until muscle exhaustion.

4. Then lower your spine and feet a bit and hold for 10 seconds.

5. Lower your legs and back to the floor.

# Level 3: High-Intensity Peak

These are the most challenging exercises and variations, but again, the previous exercises are as effective. Intensity is the key.

LEGS

## Exercise 1: Lunges

Target: *legs and butt*

1. Step forward with one leg.

2. Drop your back knee straight down until both knees are at 90 degree angles to a count of 10. Do not lunge forward. Keep your upper body straight with your shoulders back and relaxed and your chin up. Make sure your front knee is aligned over your ankle. Keep the back heel up and the toes of both feet facing forward.

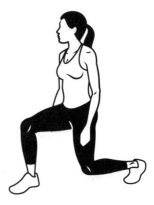

3. Rise to a standing lunge position to a count of 10 and repeat slowly until muscle exhaustion.

4. Then drop halfway down and hold for a count of 10.

## Exercise 2: One-Legged Calf Raise

Target: *lower legs*

1. Stand on a thick book, stool, chair, or step/stairs while holding on to the back of a chair or a railing. Take your right leg and hook it behind your left.

2. Keeping your body straight and eyes facing forward, raise your left heel up as far as possible to a count of 10.

3. Pause and squeeze your calf muscle, then slowly lower your heal down as far as you can to a count of 10.

4. Repeat this movement until muscle exhaustion and then switch legs.

5. Do the exercise with your other leg.

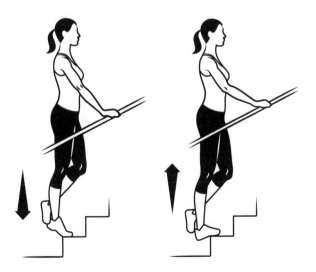

## Exercise 3: Classic Push-Up

This variation uses your feet as the pivot point.

Target: *front of shoulders, back of arms, chest, and upper back*

1. Lie down on the floor with your hands shoulder-width apart at your shoulders.

2. Rise up on your toes and hold your body in a straight line by tightening your abs to a count of 10.

3. Slowly bend your arms at the elbow and lower your body as close to the floor as you can to a count of 10. Tighten your abs and don't let your back sag. Hold your body in a straight line from your toes to the top of your head to keep your butt from pointing up in the air. Keep your head in a neutral position with your eyes down.

4. Lift your body slowly by straightening your arms to a count of 10. Remember to keep your abs tight.

5. Repeat until muscle exhaustion, then raise yourself halfway and count to 10.

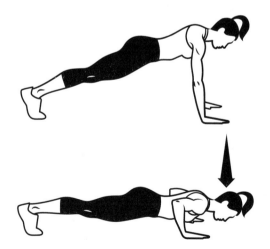

## Exercise 4: Diamond Push-Up

This push-up can be done from your knees or your toes. The change in hand position really works to intensify this exercise.

Target: *triceps*

1. Get into push-up position, move your hands together, and create a diamond with them.

2. Lower your body slowly to the floor to a count of 10, keeping your abs tight and back straight.

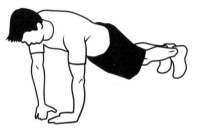

3. Lift your body to the starting position to a count of 10 and repeat the movement until muscle exhaustion.

CORE

## Exercise 5: Superman

Target: *abs and back*

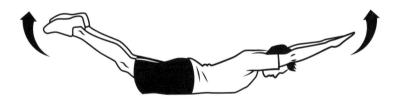

1. Lie face down on the floor with your arms stretched in front of you.

2. Slightly lift your torso and your legs at the same time to a count of 10 and pause.

3. Lower your torso and legs to a count of 10, then raise them again.

4. Repeat the exercise until muscle exhaustion.

## Exercise 6: Dynamic Prone Plank

Target: *abs, spine, and lower back*

1. Take the standard plank position.

2. Raise your hips as high as they can go to a count of 10.

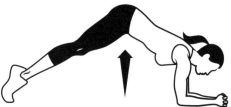

3. Lower your hips back down to a count of 10, so that your body is in a straight line and your hips don't droop.

4. Repeat the movement until muscle exhaustion.

## Exercise 7: Elevated Glute Bridge

Target: *hamstrings and butt*

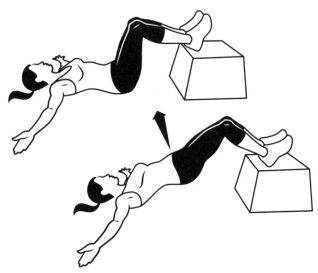

1. Lie on your back and put your feet at the ankles on a chair or a low stool.

2. Lift your spine and hips to a count of 10, keeping your abs tight and your spine straight.

3. Lower your back to the floor to a count of 10 and then lift again

4. Repeat this movement until muscle exhaustion.

## Exercise 8: Curling Up

Target: *upper and lower abs*

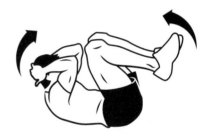

1. Lie on your back with your knees bent, feet flat, and your hands over your ears.

2. While slowly rolling up from the floor with your chin tucked, lift your knees and feet off the ground. Curl up and try to touch your knees and your elbows.

3. Hold the position until muscle exhaustion.

4. Then lower your spine and feet a bit and hold for 10 seconds.

• • •

Twenty minutes a week to do these high-intensity workouts along with moving more all day long will do so much for you. Exercise will help you break through weight loss resistance, diminish stress, alleviate depression and anxiety, improve sleep, make you look and feel younger, build calorie-burning muscle tissue, lower your risk of developing heart disease, diabetes, high blood pressure, and cancer, and reverse or improve these conditions. Exercise is a powerful medicine with impressive beneficial effects. Once you start moving, you will never want to be sedentary again. You will get a high return on your investment.

The first two parts of this book have given you the information you need to make changes in your lifestyle that will help you to lose weight. For some people, lifestyle changes alone are not enough. In Part 3, I focus on other options. Since weight control is our number-one health problem, obesity research is making great strides in developing new medications, procedures, and devices to treat this costly chronic disease. I want to answer your questions about weight loss medications and surgeries and bring you up to date on what is available and what is currently in development.

# PART 3

# Beyond Diet & Exercise

# CHAPTER 11

# Medications
# A New Frontier

If you have struggled with your weight and have yo-yo dieted for as long as you can remember, you may need more help to support your efforts. Now you understand the biological reasons for why you are having so much trouble losing those extra pounds and why your waistline is expanding. The more you try, the more your body responds by kicking into survival mode and resisting additional weight loss. A consultation with your doctor is in order if you have been doing the Change Your Biology Program for six months without success, which would be a loss of 5 to 10 percent of your body weight. Sometimes lifestyle changes are just not enough. When your health and well-being are compromised by weight loss resistance, you might need to intensify your plan. Medications are an option. In conjunction with a comprehensive program that includes changes in diet and exercise, medications have been proven to help people lose an additional 4 to 5 percent of their weight in six months.

You might consider adding medication to your weight reduction plan if your BMI is 30 or more or your BMI is 27 or more and you have one health risk factor, such as high blood pressure, high cholesterol, and/or a waist measurement of more than thirty-five inches for women and forty inches for men, and you just can't lose weight no matter what you do. You would take medication if your blood pressure or cholesterol levels were high as a matter of course. Once you consider your problem managing your weight as a chronic disease, losing weight becomes a path to improving your health. Taking medication to deal with illness is not stigmatized. Using medication for weight loss is no different. I look forward to the day when weight will be as easy to manage as high blood pressure, and I am convinced that day is not that far away.

A common misconception about weight loss medications is that simply taking a pill will make the pounds melt away magically. At the present time, weight management medications do not work on their own. You still have to make changes in your diet and move more if you want to shed pounds. Taking weight loss medication is not a cop-out or an easy way out. Medications do not cure obesity or weight problems. They have to be combined with a healthy diet and physical activity in a comprehensive program to be effective. A healthy diet may reduce injury to the neurons in the hypothalamus, which allows medication to be as effective as it can. Eating food that is calorie dense will damage the centers in your brain that the medication is designed to act on. Getting your heart rate up improves blood flow to the brain, delivering the oxygen and glucose your brain needs to function well. Exercise helps to stimulate the release of hormones that provide a nourishing environment for the growth of brain cells and stimulates the growth of new connections between brain cells. Exercise also reduces insulin resistance, which gets more fuel into the brain cells. A combination of good diet, physical activity, and medication will produce an optimal environment for correcting the source of your weight problems.

## Filling in the Gap

There has been a serious treatment gap in the way we handle chronic weight management problems. On one end of the spectrum, we use weight loss programs that involve changes in diet and exercise. It is clear that for some people, lifestyle programs are not enough to produce permanent weight loss. At the other end of the severity spectrum, surgery seems too risky to many. Medication and new minimally invasive procedures can fill that gap. Unfortunately, the growing obesity epidemic has outstripped the development of medications to help handle the difficulty people were having to control their weight, because we've spent all our time blaming people for being obese and not focusing on why it might be so hard to lose weight. Between 1999 and 2012, the Food and Drug Administration had not approved any new medications for weight management. This chart illustrates where we were in 2012.

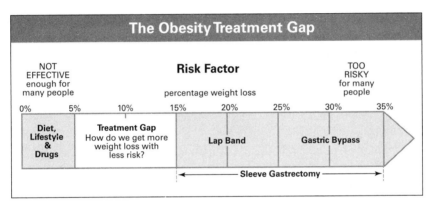

The challenge of dealing with the obesity epidemic has made discovering noninvasive ways to treat weight problems an urgent necessity. Since 2012, the FDA has approved four new medications. Pharmaceutical companies are now beginning to focus research resources on developing new, safe, and effective medications to help people who are overweight or obese overcome the biological processes that prevent them from achieving their weight goals.

Prior to 2012, the last weight loss medication to be approved by the FDA for long-term use was orlistat (brand names Xenical, Alli) in 1999. Alli is the over-the-counter form of this medication, which contains half the doses of prescription Xenical. Orlistat promotes weight loss by decreasing the amount of fat absorbed in the gastrointestinal tract by 30 percent. Though orlistat was an effective medication, it was not widely used because of gastrointestinal side effects and limited weight loss for those who took it.

Claire, who was depressed and anxious, first came to the Comprehensive Weight Control Center when she was seventeen with a BMI of 40. She had gone from 110 pounds to 150 in fourteen months and was now up to 212 pounds. She had been taking progesterone because polycystic ovarian syndrome (PCOS) had made her periods very irregular. She had low thyroid and was also taking the antidepressant Elavil, which can cause weight gain. The combination of medical conditions and medications had been a disaster for her weight. She confessed that she was a binger — ice cream, junk food, and pizza were her binge foods of choice.

When I asked her if she had tried to lose weight, she told me she had recently tried Weight Watchers without success. Her response to my question about how many diets she had tried before that was "too many." Among the diets that had not worked for her was the hCG diet, for which she injected herself with a hormone produced by pregnant women, accompanied by eating only five hundred calories a day. She claimed that she had stopped gaining weight but did not lose a pound on that extreme regimen.

At the time of her first visit, Claire was following a low-fat diet. Typically, she would start the day with reduced fat peanut butter on a 100-calorie mini bagel, half a banana, and iced coffee with skim milk. For lunch she'd have a salad with grilled chicken dressed with balsamic vinegar or lemon. Her main meal was grilled chicken with brown rice and a green salad, diet Snapple, with an apple and nuts for an evening snack. Low fat was not working for her at all. She claimed never to be satiated with "healthy food" and craved french fries, sweets, chocolate, and pizza. We explained to Claire that adding some fat to her diet and more vegetables would help her to feel more full and satisfied.

I gave her a prescription for metformin and a small dose of phentermine, half a pill a day. She started to lose weight. After a year, she was down to 175 pounds, a little over a 10 percent weight loss. To treat her migraines, I added Topamax to her medications. She went on to lose an additional fourteen pounds the next year, which put her at 161 pounds. She stopped taking metformin and began to eat carbs and her weight went up to 165, so she resumed taking that medication.

She went off to college, stopped taking her medications, ate like a typical college freshman away from home, and added alcohol to the mix. After four months, she was up to 190.8 pounds. She came to the office during her holiday break and left determined to take her medications again. She lost seven pounds during her three-week Christmas break, but had trouble keeping the weight off once she got back to school, and finished the year weighing 190 pounds.

Claire was more motivated her sophomore year. We adjusted her medication and by the end of the academic year, she was down to 155.6 pounds, a forty-pound weight loss. Two things were different: she started to exercise, and she fell in love.

She began eating smaller meals and continued to work out while taking the same medications. Her weight went down to 134.6 during the summer.

In her junior year, she had some issues and began to take Adderall instead of her phentermine each day. She maintained her weight. When she started her senior year, she stopped taking Topamax and started Zoloft. Her weight went up to 139. Claire had learned that she had to catch it as soon as she saw her weight going in the wrong direction. She started to exercise more, and by the time she graduated was down to 133 pounds. She had trouble finding a job and was overqualified for the job she finally landed. She decreased her exercise and was less conscious about what she was eating. Her weight was up to 142 pounds by the holidays.

When she came in to see me, we looked at her medications and revised the list. Her new regimen included metformin, Zoloft, and Qsymia, which had just been approved by the FDA. Six weeks later she had lost six pounds and was down to 136. She has managed to maintain her weight by paying attention when she begins to gain. She now knows what she has to do to stop her weight from climbing.

I have related this lengthy history, which spans five years, so that you will be aware that while there are sometimes many ups and downs when you try to lose weight, you cannot give up. You are dealing with your body's natural inclination to store energy for hard times—but you can outsmart that drive. There is always something else you can try—an adjustment in medication, exercising more, being more rigorous about your diet—to get back on track. You have to take a long view, stay focused, and keep your goals in mind. If you stray from the path, get right back on it.

The thinking used to be that weight loss medications needed to be taken for only a few months. Phentermine, which first appeared in 1959, is one of four noradrenergic drugs, including diethylpropion, benzphetamine, and phendinetrazine, approved by the FDA for short-term use. These drugs amplify the transmission of nerve impulses from norepinephrine, a hormone and neurotransmitter. The medications promote weight loss by activating the sympathetic nervous system. Working on the hypothalamus, phentermine increases resting energy expenditure and decreases food intake. The drugs could cause increased heart rate and blood pressure in some people, and they haven't been studied over the long term, which is why their use has been restricted to short term. Weight loss appears to be greatest during the first weeks with these drugs, but a plateau ensues after three to six months in most patients. In the past, it was thought the effect of the medicine had worn off, or the patient lost willpower. Now we know that it is the result of compensation elsewhere in the weight-regulating systems of the body. And that is a treatable problem.

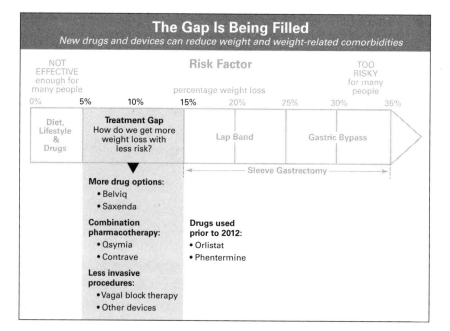

Now that obesity is considered a chronic disease and regaining weight after dieting is recognized as a problem of neurologic and metabolic weight-regulating mechanisms, the new medications are designed for long-term weight maintenance. The drugs reinforce changes in diet by helping to reduce appetite and food intake. The new medications help patients to stick to their diet programs. Weight is often regained when the medication is stopped. Just as you would take your diabetes medication to regulate your illness, for most people these medications have to be taken daily to control a chronic condition.

## The Latest Developments

With four new drugs on the market at the beginning of 2015, I want to introduce you to the newest medications now available. I discuss their properties, positive effects, possible side effects, and whether the medication could be harmful to you if you have certain conditions or are taking other medications that will interact badly. I also recommend who would benefit most from each medication. This background will prepare you for a conversation with your health care provider about whether weight loss medications are a good plan of action for you and, if so, which medication would be most beneficial.

### Lorcaserin (Belviq)
### Dose: 10 mg twice daily

Approved in 2012, Belviq controls appetite by activating the serotonin receptors in the brain. The neurotransmitter serotonin triggers feelings of satiety and satisfaction and is associated with mood. This medication is designed to stimulate only one type of serotonin receptor, the 2C receptor, in the appetite center of the brain and not in other areas of the brain or the body. In the 1990s, heart valve problems and a very rare problem called pulmonary hypertension were seen with older serotonin medications, which hit several recep-tors and affected heart valves. This has not been seen in the trials of Belviq after careful evaluation of the heart in several thousand people. Nonetheless, additional long-term studies are ongoing to be absolutely certain. Caution has to be observed in combining Belviq with other drugs that affect serotonin neurotransmitters like the cat-egory of antidepressants called serotonin reuptake inhibitors (SSRIs). Your doctor should review a complete list of all the medications and supplements you are taking before prescribing this medication for you. Belviq seems to work particularly well in some people, and not in others. As a result, if you don't lose 5 percent of your body weight after twelve weeks of taking Belviq, you should stop taking the drug, because using the medication for a longer time is not likely to lead to significant weight loss. Those who lose 5 percent after twelve weeks go on to lose on average 10 percent of their body weight, a great, medically significant result. As I've mentioned, adding medicine, not increasing it, can give additional weight loss. In the first study look-ing at this, taking Belviq along with phentermine, which works in a different way, was shown to double weight loss compared to taking Belviq alone.

Positive Effects: The benefits of weight loss, including decreased blood pressure, heart rate, blood sugar, and other risk factors as weight is lost.

Possible Side Effects: Headache, dizziness, fatigue, nausea, dry mouth, constipation, and in patients with diabetes, low blood sugar if you are taking other medications to lower your sugar.

Not recommended for: People with valvular heart disease, those taking drugs for valvular heart disease, certain drugs for depression, migraine, mood, anxiety, psychotic, or thought disorders, including triptans, MAOIs, SSRIs, SNRIs, tricyclic antidepressants; anyone with kidney or liver disease, sickle cell anemia, multiple myeloma or leukemia; pregnant women.

Phentermine/Topiramate (Qsymia)
Dose: phentermine 3.75 mg/topiramate
23 mg; 7.5 mg/46 mg; 15 mg/92 mg

This combination drug, approved in 2012, has produced the highest percentage of body weight loss in comparison with the other new weight loss medications because it combines two effective medicines into one pill. Qsymia contains low doses of these medications in a controlled-release form to minimize side effects. The dose of both drugs is smaller than typically used. Since the dose of phentermine in this combination drug is so low (one-eighth of maximum), the risks formerly associated with taking phentermine are reduced. Phentermine is an appetite suppressant and topiramate is an anticonvulsant, which prevents migraines. Topiramate helps to reduce body weight by several mechanisms including reducing food intake as well as increasing fat cell metabolism. It is clear that this medication combines the effects of topiramate with those of phentermine.

**Positive Effects:** The benefits of weight loss, including decreased blood pressure, blood sugar, and other risk factors as weight is lost. Shown to reduce triglycerides, increase HDL (good) cholesterol, improve insulin levels, reduce levels of inflammatory hormones, and reduce the progression to type 2 diabetes.

**Possible Side Effects:** Increase in heart rate, a sensation of numbness in the fingers or toes known as paresthesias, dizziness, dry mouth, insomnia, anxiety, mood changes such as feeling depressed, and difficulty concentrating.

**Not recommended for:** Anyone with a history of cardiac problems, coronary disease, uncontrolled hypertension, hyperthyroidism, or glaucoma. Since this medication can increase the risk of developing kidney stones, you should be cautious if you have a history of this condition. Do not take this medication if you have taken an MAO inhibitor within fourteen days. Though pregnant women should not take any weight loss medication, it is particularly important to have a pregnancy test before taking this medication if you are trying to get pregnant or could possibly be pregnant, because it increases the risk of the fetus developing a cleft palate when taken during the first trimester.

### Bupropion/naltrexone (Contrave)
### Dose: 90 mg/ 8 mg tablets

|        | Morning Dose | Evening Dose |
|--------|--------------|--------------|
| Week 1 | 1 tablet     | none         |
| Week 2 | 1 tablet     | 1 tablet     |
| Week 3 | 2 tablets    | 1 tablet     |
| Week 4 | 2 tablets    | 2 tablets    |

We start Contrave at 1 tablet daily and increase weekly or even more gradually if weight loss occurs. We often stop at a lower dose if getting a good effect to minimize side effects and increase as needed to the maximum.

The FDA approved Contrave in 2014. It combines bupropion, which is used to treat depression and seasonal affective disorder, and as an aid to smoking cessation. Bupropion inhibits the reabsorption of dopamine and norepinephrine in the brain, leading to enhancement of the reward pathway that food can induce, thus reducing the drive to eat. Naltrexone is used to treat alcohol and opioid dependence. In this case, it blocks an opioid pathway that may reduce the effectiveness of bupropion at reducing food intake.

**Positive Effects:** The benefits of weight loss, including decreased blood pressure and blood sugar and improvement in other risk factors as weight is lost.

**Possible Side Effects:** Nausea and vomiting, constipation, headache, dizziness, insomnia, dry mouth, diarrhea, elevated blood pressure and heart rate in some patients, seizure, anxiety.

**Not recommended for:** Anyone with uncontrolled hypertension, a seizure disorder, an eating disorder, narcotic addiction or taking medication to treat one, dependent on opioid pain medicines or with chronic pain (can increase pain sensitivity), using other medications that contain bupropion such as Wellbutrin, Wellbutrin SR, Wellbutrin XL, Aplenzin, and Zyban, use sedatives or anti-seizure medication, who has taken MAOIs in the past fourteen days, are pregnant or planning to become pregnant.

---

### Liraglutide (Saxenda)
### Dose: 0.6–3.0 mg daily by subcutaneous injection

---

Saxenda was approved by the FDA as a treatment for diabetes in 2010. The FDA approved a higher dose for the treatment of obesity in late 2014. It is the only weight management medication that requires subcutaneous injection. The drug mimics the effect of GLP-1, an intestinal hormone that suppresses appetite, increases satiety, and delays the emptying of the stomach. In patients with diabetes, it augments insulin release and reduces blood sugar. The dose of Saxenda starts low at 0.6 mg daily and is titrated up gradually, on a weekly basis. We often stop at a lower dose if we are getting a good effect.

**Positive Effects:** The benefits of weight loss, including reduced blood pressure, blood sugar, waist circumference, reduced risk of developing diabetes, and lower triglyceride and LDL (bad) cholesterol levels.

**Possible Side Effects:** Headache, nausea, vomiting, fatigue, dizziness, abdominal pain, constipation, increased pulse rate, increased risk of gallstones and inflammation of the pancreas (rare).

**Not Recommended for:** People with a personal or family history of thyroid cancer or the rare, inherited disorder of multiple endocrine neoplasia, in which several endocrine glands develop benign or malignant tumors, pancreatitis.

### Phentermine
### Dose: 18.75–37.5 mg once daily

Phentermine reduces appetite. It is the most widely prescribed weight loss medication in the United States. Available since 1959, it is approved for three month use, but is often used over a longer period of time, known as "off-label" prescribing. When we use phentermine it is usually at lower doses such as ¼ or ½ tablet to minimize side effects.

**Positive Effects:** The benefits of weight loss, including decreased blood pressure, blood sugar, and other risk factors as weight is lost. Shown to reduce triglycerides and increase HDL (good) cholesterol.

**Possible Side Effects:** Increase in heart rate and blood pressure, dizziness, dry mouth, insomnia, anxiety. Mood changes such as feeling depressed.

**Not Recommended for:** Anyone with a history of cardiac problems, coronary disease, uncontrolled hypertension, hyperthyroidism, or glaucoma. Do not take this medication if you have taken an MAO inhibitor within fourteen days. Pregnant women.

Metformin (Glucophage)
Dose: 500 mg to start, up to 1000 mg twice daily

Another medication we often use in patients with prediabetes or those who have signs of insulin resistance is metformin, the most widely used medication for the treatment of type 2 diabetes. This is known as "off-label" prescribing, because even though the patient doesn't have diabetes, studies have shown that using metformin reduces the risk of developing diabetes by more than 30 percent. It may have other medical benefits as well, including reducing the risk of heart disease and certain cancers.

Designed to help a person with diabetes control his blood sugar, metformin is believed to have many mechanisms of action, appearing indirectly to reverse insulin resistance and make the brain more sensitive to leptin. In my opinion, metformin should be approved as a weight loss medication.

**Positive Effects:** The benefits of weight loss, including reduced blood pressure, blood sugar, waist circumference, risk of developing diabetes, and lower triglyceride and LDL levels.

**Possible Side Effects:** Headache, nausea, muscle aches, diarrhea or constipation.

**Not Recommended for:** People with congestive heart, kidney, or liver failure, because metformin can cause a life-threatening condition called lactic acidosis.

**Recommended for:** People with type 2 diabetes, prediabetes, insulin resistance, polycystic ovarian syndrome (PCOS).

We are filling the gap in the middle of the treatment spectrum with new and effective medications. Think of medical treatment before antibiotics were developed. Millions of people suffered and lost their lives because their illnesses could not be treated successfully. Now we take antibiotics for granted. A broad selection of antibiotics exists with medications targeted to specific conditions. I expect the same progress with weight loss medications. We have already started to create medications that effectively treat our number-one health care problem. Those medications will only become more sophisticated and their use commonplace and universally accepted.

•   •   •

The other frontier in the fight against obesity is surgical procedures. For many of my patients with severe obesity, bariatric surgery is a means to achieving the weight loss that has eluded them despite trying their various programs and medications. When their bodies are strongly resistant to losing weight, they are relieved to know that surgery can help them. The following chapter will explain the surgeries available now, the newest approved obesity treatment devices, and the realities of the day-to-day consequences of having bariatric surgery.

# CHAPTER 12

# The Surgical Solution for Severe Obesity

AS WEIGHT SHIFTS HIGHER GLOBALLY, the most dramatic increase has been in the steep rise in the rates of severe obesity, which is determined by a BMI of 40 or more. In the past thirty years, severe obesity has increased 350 percent in the United States. Recent studies have found that death rates in adults with severe obesity are about 2.5 times higher than in adults in the normal weight range. According to other studies, having severe obesity can cut 6.5 to 13.7 years off your life. Although most people can lose weight and dramatically improve their health with diet, exercise, and medication, some need surgery to control their weight. My patients with severe obesity could not be more motivated to lose weight. They have tried everything—many different weight loss plans and medications—without lasting success. Their weight will not drop significantly no matter what they do, and they often have health complications. In their frustration, they are ready to do anything and are open to consider surgery as a last resort. We used to think that weight loss surgeries made changes to your digestive system to help you lose weight by limiting the amount you eat and/or reducing the nutrients you absorb. We now know that is an oversimplification of the facts. Research is showing that there are multiple changes in body weight–regulating mechanisms, including changes to hormones that control weight and the bacteria found in the intestine, the microbiome, that can contribute to weight loss. Even the vagus nerve has been studied. The newest approved obesity treatment device, the first in ten years, targets the vagus nerve with a device that is implanted into the abdomen.

When it comes to surgery, I spend time educating my patients about the next step they are thinking of taking. They have to be well informed about the benefits and risks of surgery, the different procedures, and the long-term effects they can expect. These surgeries are major, life-changing procedures. Choosing to have surgery is a big step, but one that is well worth the risk for most. Though surgery always carries risks, like many things in life, the greater the risk, the greater the potential benefit in terms of pounds lost and health benefit.

In the end, the long-term success of these procedures depends on your ability to make permanent changes in your lifestyle. Bariatric surgery is not a quick fix. These surgeries are tools that will help you control hunger and portion size, but the rest is up to you. Eating "fattening" foods minimizes the amount you can lose with surgery, while eating "healthy" food can maximize it.

A team of professionals should support your efforts to adapt your eating and lifestyle habits following surgery. If postoperative support is not available, it is my opinion that you may be in the wrong place. I would recommend you seek your surgery someplace else.

### YOU ARE A CANDIDATE FOR SURGERY IF:

- you have a BMI of 40 or higher.

- you have a BMI of 35 or higher and have serious weight-related complications like sleep apnea or diabetes, and other methods of treatment have failed.

*Or*

- you are 50 to 100 percent above your ideal body weight.

- you are 100 pounds or more overweight.

If you want to reduce surgical risk, I advise you to go to a busy center, preferably one that specializes in obesity management. The multidisciplinary teams at these specialized centers have experience in assessing patients before surgery, doing the procedures, and diagnosing and managing complications. The surgeons and the centers have established a good track record and offer excellent long-term follow-up care. An aftercare program that focuses on dietary, exercise, and behavioral changes is very important. Your success depends in large part on your working with the center you chose to change your lifestyle. To find centers of excellence for surgery, check the programs that have met the American College of Surgeons Metabolic and Bariatric Surgery quality standards at

https://www.facs.org/search/bariatric-surgery-centers

The American Society for Metabolic and Bariatric Surgery lists its members at https://asmbs.org/patients/find-a-provider.

# Bariatric Surgery Procedures

Most bariatric procedures are minimally invasive and use laparoscopic surgery. A review of the most commonly performed procedures follows.

### THE LAPAROSCOPIC SLEEVE GASTRECTOMY

The most commonly performed surgical procedure, the sleeve gastrectomy, or gastric sleeve, reduces the size of your stomach. The minimally invasive procedure removes about 80 percent of the stomach, making the stomach approximately the size and shape of a banana. Reducing the volume of the stomach and changing its shape causes food to get to the duodenum, the first section of the intestine, more rapidly.

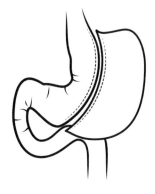

Laparoscopic sleeve gastrectomy

Rob came to us about four years ago. He was in his late thirties and struggling. He was taking medication for his depression. His weight kept going
up. He had type 2 diabetes and very high triglycerides and LDL cholesterol.
When he hit 276 pounds, he knew he had to do something before his health
got worse. He came to see me, determined to do what he could to take
control of his weight and his health. His BMI was 38.5, and he already had
metabolic syndrome.

This first thing I did was to change his medications and to put him
on the Quick Start Change Your Biology Diet. He was on insulin, Symlin,
and metformin to control his diabetes and weight. He stuck to it and lost
weight steadily. When he weighed in at 227 pounds, forty-nine pounds
lighter than he had been when he started, his weight loss slowed down. He
had lost almost 18 percent of his body weight over a two-year period. Rob's
numbers had improved and his spirits were higher, but he had diabetes and
wanted to lose more.

We talked about what a reasonable next step would be for him. In our
discussion of bariatric surgery, I pointed out that a sleeve gastrectomy was
the least invasive surgery he could have and the recuperation would be
the quickest. Confident that he could get his weight down, he decided to
have the surgery. The procedure went well with a great outcome. By the
time he had the surgery, his weight had climbed back up to 253 pounds.
Six months after surgery, he had dropped an additional forty-two pounds.
He was down to 185 pounds. He has lost a total of ninety-one pounds — a
little more than 35 percent of his original weight — and has maintained
most of the weight loss. Rob is a different person than the young man
I first met. His health has improved, and his sugars are normal. He has
grown to know himself well. He has learned to recognize and deal with
his emotional problems by heading them off at the pass. Being so much
lighter has made physical activity easier. He started to practice martial
arts, which has boosted his energy and optimism. He is an upbeat, fit man
at forty-three. He is one of my most enthusiastic patients.

That leads to higher levels of GLP-1, a gut hormone that reduces appetite and lowers blood sugar.

In addition, the surgery removes the part of the stomach that produces the gut hormone ghrelin, which normally increases your appetite before a meal. This helps to explain why this surgery has been so effective: many changes that reduce body weight occur at the same time.

This procedure does not require implanting a band around a portion of the stomach as gastric banding does. Sleeve gastrectomy is a simpler operation than gastric bypass, because it doesn't involve rerouting or reconnecting the intestines. The procedure can be performed as part of a two-step process for patients with a BMI over 60. The sleeve is performed first to allow the patient to lose enough weight so that a bypass can be performed with much lower health risks.

## POSITIVES

- Restricts the amount of food the stomach can hold.

- Causes favorable changes in gut hormones that reduce appetite and suppress hunger.

- Weight loss is faster than with gastric banding.

- On average, 25 percent of body weight is lost.

- Requires no implantable band device, no risk of slippage and erosion, and has a simpler follow-up than banding.

- There is no bypass or rerouting of the food stream.

- Surgical risk is lower than with gastric bypass procedures.

- The minimally invasive techniques speed recovery time to approximately two days.

## NEGATIVES

- The procedure is not reversible.

- Weight loss is somewhat less than gastric bypass.

- It has the potential for vitamin deficiencies.

- Complications are slightly higher than with gastric banding.

### COMPLICATIONS

- Standard surgical risks

- Blood clots

- Leakage at site of sutures

### TIMELINE FOR RECOVERY

- Two day average hospital stay

- Return to normal activity in two weeks for most patients

- Full surgical recovery usually by three weeks

## *State of the Art*

I do want to mention a new procedure we are working on — the endoscopic gastroplasty sleeve. This procedure is less invasive than the gastric sleeve, because the sewing is done from inside the gastrointestinal system by going endoscopically through the mouth. More work needs to be done, but the results are promising. While not as effective as the surgical gastroplasty, it is even less invasive and is done as an outpatient procedure.

### ADJUSTABLE GASTRIC BAND

This procedure, popularly called the "lap band," involves placing an inflatable band around the upper part of the stomach. No cutting or stapling is needed to separate the upper stomach pouch from the lower stomach. The small stomach pouch created above the band restricts the amount of food that can be consumed at one time. The band also increases the time it takes for the stomach to empty. The size of the opening between the pouch and the remainder of the stomach created by the gastric band determines how long it takes your stomach to empty, making you feel full longer. The size of the stomach opening can be adjusted by filling the band with sterile saline, which is injected through a port placed under the skin. Reducing the size of the opening is done gradually over time with adjustments, or "fills," as they are called.

When performing gastric banding surgery, the surgeon makes a few small incisions in the abdominal wall. The ad-

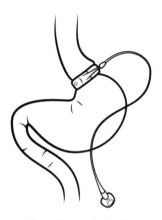

Adjustable gastric band

justable silicone band is inserted and secured around the upper part of the stomach using laparoscopic techniques. The band is connected to tubing, which attaches to an access port fixed beneath the skin of the abdomen. The port, used to make adjustments in the band, is under the skin and can only be felt by pushing on the abdomen. The procedure takes about forty minutes and for most people can be performed on an outpatient basis with no hospital stay required.

The band has been considered a restrictive procedure, because it limits how much food you can eat at each meal and restricts the emptying of the stomach pouch through the band. Studies have challenged this assumption by showing that food passes through the band quickly and concluding that reduced hunger and increased satiety is not related to the food that remained in the pouch above the band. There is no malabsorption. Food is digested and absorbed as it is normally.

## POSITIVES

- Reduces the amount of food the stomach can hold.

- Creates a physical sense of fullness, possibly because it may compress the vagus nerve.

- Involves no cutting of the stomach or rerouting of intestines.

- Patients lose an average of 17 to 20 percent of their excess weight.

- Some centers do the surgery on an outpatient basis. If not, the hospital stay is usually less than twenty-four hours.

- The procedure is reversible and adjustable.

- Has the lowest rate of early postoperative complications among approved bariatric procedures.

- Has the lowest risk for vitamin/mineral deficiencies.

### NEGATIVES

- Slower and less early weight loss than other surgical procedures.

- Less effective than other techniques in weight loss and maintaining loss.

- A foreign device remains in the body.

- Band slippage or band erosion into the stomach occurs in a small percentage of patients.

- Possible mechanical problems with the band, tube, or port.

- Overeating can cause dilation of the esophagus.

- Requires strict adherence to postoperative follow-up visits and diet.

- Highest rate of reoperation.

## ROUX-EN-Y GASTRIC BYPASS
### (MINIMALLY INVASIVE)

The Roux-en-Y gastric bypass is named after the surgeon who began using the procedure and the two branches it forms in the small intestine. With this type of bypass, a small pouch is created at the top of the stomach using surgical staples. The pouch is about the size of an egg. The next component of the surgery involves the small intestine. The first portion of the small intestine is divided and the bottom end of the divided small intestine is brought up and connected to the new stomach pouch with staples. The procedure is completed by connecting the top portion of the divided small intestine to the small intestine farther down so that the stomach acids and digestive enzymes from the bypassed stomach and first portion of small intestine will mix with the food eventually. This procedure bypasses the part of the stomach that is mainly responsible for digesting food, and part of the intestines.

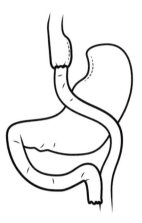

Roux-en-Y gastric bypass

The small stomach pouch results in consuming smaller meals, but much more is going on in the bypass than that. Most important is that rerouting the food stream produces changes in gut hormones that promote satiety, suppress hunger, and improve insulin sensitivity, reversing one of the main mechanisms that results in obesity-induced type 2 diabetes. Recent research on the bypass shows that even the intestinal bacteria changes in a way that promotes weight loss! Normally, when you go on a diet, intestinal bacteria appear, to resist weight loss but with gastric bypass, the change in microbiome appears to contribute to greater weight loss.

## POSITIVES

- Restricts the amount of food that can be consumed.

- Rapid initial weight loss.

- Produces an average 30 to 35 percent body weight loss.

- Longest clinical experience of any surgery.

- Rapid improvement or resolution of type 2 diabetes and metabolic syndrome.

- Favorable changes in gut hormones to reduce hunger and enhance satiety.

## NEGATIVES

- Cutting and stapling of the stomach and intestines are required.

- A more complex operation than the band or gastric sleeve, with potentially greater complication rates.

- Portion of digestive tract is bypassed, which can lead to vitamin and mineral deficiencies, particularly vitamin B12, thiamine, iron, calcium, and folate.

- Dumping syndrome or rapid gastric emptying can occur. When the undigested contents of your stomach, usually starch or sugar, move too rapidly into your small bowel, you can develop stomach cramps, nausea, and diarrhea. Most people with dumping syndrome experience symptoms soon after eating, while others have late symptoms that occur one to three hours after eating. Some people experience both early and late symptoms.

- The procedure is not adjustable and is difficult to reverse.

- Slightly higher mortality rate, in the range of gall bladder surgery.

### COMPLICATIONS

- Standard risks associated with surgery, more common than with other procedures.

- Up to 5% percent of patients experience significant complications, other complications are more common than with other procedures.

- Leaks from staple lines, requiring revisional surgery.

### RECOVERY TIME

- Hospital stay, usually two or three days.

- Many patients return to normal activity within two and a half weeks.

- Full surgical recovery usually within three weeks.

## Bariatric Surgeries Compared

For easy reference, this chart gives you an overview of weight loss surgeries. Each surgical procedure has its own benefits and risks, which you need to evaluate with your doctor.

## Sleeve Gastrectomy

| | |
|---|---|
| Description of Procedure | A thin vertical sleeve of stomach, about the size of a banana, is created using a stapling device. The rest of the stomach is removed. |
| How It Contributes to Weight Loss | The sleeve, a smaller stomach pouch, causes food to get to the duodenum, which produces a gut hormone that reduces appetite and lowers blood sugar. The procedure removes the part of the stomach that produces the gut hormone which increases appetite. Limits how much food can be consumed at one time, resulting in feeling full sooner and staying full longer. Since your calorie intake is reduced, your body uses its fat for energy. |
| How Digestion Is Affected | Food passes through the digestive tract in the usual order and is fully absorbed in the body. |
| Total Body Weight Loss | 25% |

### Health Benefits *(Shown in Clinical Trials)*

| | |
|---|---|
| Type 2 Diabetes | 45 to 58% medication no longer needed |
| High Blood Pressure | 50% medication no longer needed |
| Obstructive Sleep Apnea | 60% medication no longer needed |
| Procedures Performed in 2014 | 104,220 |

| Gastric Band | Gastric Bypass |
|---|---|
| An inflatable band is wrapped around the upper part of the stomach, dividing the stomach in a small upper pouch that holds about ½ cup of food and a larger lower stomach. The degree of band tightness affects how much food can be consumed and the length of time it takes for food to leave the stomach pouch. | The surgeon creates a small stomach pouch and attaches a section of the small intestine directly to the pouch, allowing food to bypass a portion of the small intestine. |
| The band severely restricts the amount of food that can be eaten at one time, because it creates a smaller stomach pouch. You feel full sooner and stay full longer. | A gastric bypass, like the sleeve and the band, creates a smaller stomach pouch that limits how much food can be eaten at one time.<br><br>By rerouting the food stream, changes occur in gut hormones that promote satiety, suppress hunger, and improve insulin sensitivity. There are changes in the gut microbiome that promote weight loss as well. |
| Does not significantly affect normal digestion and absorption. Food is fully absorbed. | Reduces the amount of nutrients absorbed. |
| 20% | 33% |
| 20 to 59% | 60 to 84% |
| 42% medication no longer needed | 66% medication no longer needed |
| 45% medication no longer needed | 76% medication no longer needed |
| 15,440 | 46,320 |

Now that you are familiar with the procedures used today, you may decide to pursue the option of weight loss surgery. For many people, bariatric surgery not only spurs significant weight loss but improves or eliminates serious health problems, enhances quality of life, and extends life expectancy by years. Before you commit to surgery, it helps to know how your life will change as a result. You will be in for many changes you might not expect.

## What to Expect Post-Surgery

During the first three to six months following surgery, you will be losing weight rapidly. Most people feel better than ever. It is important to eat protein and take vitamins and minerals during this time.

Gallstones are common when you lose a significant amount of weight quickly. Up to 10 percent of gastric bypass patients develop gallstones after surgery, which can cause nausea, vomiting, and abdominal pain. Your doctor may give you a medicine called ursodiol to help prevent the stones. It works, so if your doctor prescribes it, take it.

After you lose so much weight, your body shape and contour will obviously change. The change may result in saggy skin and loss of muscle mass. The more weight you lose, the more excess skin you might have. Loose skin tends to occur most commonly around the belly, thighs, buttocks, and upper arms, as well as your chest, neck, and face. Exercise is important before and after surgery. Strength training, like the workouts in Chapter 10, will shape and tone the muscles that support your skin. Your physician will guide you on the best way to handle excess skin. Some patients elect to have plastic surgery to remove loose skin.

## How Your Eating Will Change

You might be wondering how you will eat after your stomach has been reduced to a small pouch the size of an egg or a banana. For two to three weeks after surgery, you will eat liquid or pureed foods only. You will gradually add soft foods and then normal solid foods to your diet. By six weeks, your diet will consist of normal food.

Once you are eating solid food, each bite must be chewed twenty to thirty times. The food you eat has to be smooth or pureed before you swallow it. It is important to wait two to three minutes after swallowing before putting the next bite of food in your mouth. This is very important, because if you have a band or bypass, the opening of your new stomach will be very small and food that is not chewed well can block the opening, causing you to vomit or feel pain under your breastbone. Since you have to chew your food completely and pause between bites, each meal will take at least a half hour or longer. Instead of eating three meals a day, you will be eating six small meals. Some foods may cause you discomfort if they are not chewed very well, including raw vegetables; meats; dry, sticky, or stringy foods; pasta; rice; and bread.

It is important to drink up to eight glasses of water or other calorie-free liquids every day. You need to take small sips. Avoid straws, because they bring air into your stomach. Do not drink while you are eating or for an hour before or after you eat. If you do, you may feel full before you have eaten enough food. Having liquid in your stomach will wash food out and make you hungry.

You will feel full very quickly at first, often after only a few bites of solid food, because just after surgery your new stomach pouch will only hold a tablespoon of food. A normal stomach holds up to 4 cups of food. Even after the pouch expands, it will not hold more than a cup of chewed food.

Following a healthy diet plan remains important. Your meals should be composed of vegetables, protein, fruit, and some whole grains, just as you eat on the Change Your Biology Diet, to support weight loss. You will not be eating foods full of sugar, starch, or fat or drinks that contain high-fructose corn syrup or sugar. If you eat or drink foods high in sugar, particularly sodas and fruit juices, dumping syndrome can occur. The sugary food rushes through the stomach and can cause nausea, vomiting, and weakness. The bubbles in carbonated drinks could make you uncomfortable. You should avoid

Nora, fifty-three, had been overweight for years. She had tried every popular fad diet and always regained the weight. She has a big job at a foundation and travels the world for humanitarian missions and conferences. Her lowest weight as an adult had been 165 pounds, her high 250+. She had been taking Provera, a medication associated with weight gain, to alleviate menopausal symptoms. She refused bariatric surgery for personal reasons. I worked with her gynecologist to prescribe a hormone replacement therapy that minimized weight gain. Over time, we tried different weight loss medications. She made lifestyle changes and was losing weight, but plateaued at a higher weight than we wanted. Nora decided to try the new endoscopic sleeve gastroplasty, which our gastroenterologists were developing at the time. She had the procedure on a Tuesday and was playing tennis by Friday. She weighed 215 pounds with a BMI of 34.7 when she had the procedure. In six months, she was down to 181 pounds with a BMI of 29.2. She reported that she would still get hungry, but was able to be satisfied with much less food.

To help her avoid regaining weight, she takes metformin, bupropion, and phentermine. She eats carefully and does work some protein shakes into her diet. Given the amount of time she spends sitting on airplanes and at conferences, she has an exercise routine that she does faithfully wherever she is in the world. She has found that exercise helps her to maintain her weight loss.

the empty calories of alcoholic beverages. Over time, drinking more alcohol is a problem that some patients have after bariatric surgery. It's important to make your medical team aware of this problem if you notice it.

# Reality vs. Expectations

Some patients feel blue after surgery. The optimistic belief that everything was going to be easier after surgery might be shaken by the recovery, the follow-up visits, and the continued attention to diet and exercise necessary to drop weight. The reality of life after surgery may be different from what you expected. Habits, attitudes, feelings, and concerns you thought would change might still exist. For example, you might have hoped that you would not miss food after surgery, that your cravings for high-calorie foods would no longer trouble you, only to find that the cravings are still there. You might underestimate how much you would miss social rituals that revolve around food such as eating out or celebrating with friends. You can still do these things, but what and how you eat will be different. They way friends and family react to your weight loss and post-surgery lifestyle may not be as enthusiastic and supportive as you had hoped. And weight loss might not relieve you of self-doubt and anxiety. Losing weight might have seemed to be the answer to all your problems, but you might find it is just a beginning to dealing with them. A period of adjustment is necessary on your path to controlling your weight. You will adapt to your new normal and come to appreciate the changes you have worked so hard to accomplish.

# New Devices

Several new treatments for obesity are not yet available in the United States as of this writing but are worth mentioning here. They are the Maestro Rechargeable System, which focuses on the vagus nerve, the intragastric balloon, which is inflated in the stomach and increases fullness, the Aspire Assist, which allows patients to remove food from their stomachs, and GI Dynamics EndoBarrier, which involves lining parts of the intestine. Clinical trials are now being run for these treatments.

### vBLOC MAESTRO SYSTEM

In January 2015, the FDA approved an electrical stimulation device for treating obesity that targets the abdominal vagus nerve. This is the first weight loss treatment device that targets the nerve pathway between the brain and the stomach that controls feelings of hunger and fullness. The device consists of a rechargeable electrical pulse generator, wire leads, and electrodes that are surgically implanted into the abdomen. External controls allow the patient to charge the device and health care professionals to adjust the device's settings to provide optimal therapy and minimize side effects.

The device is implanted under the skin of the torso just like a pacemaker. Instead of going to the heart, the device's leads wrap around both branches of the vagus nerve near the stomach. The vBloc Maestro sends electrical pulses to the two branches of the abdominal vagus nerve, which regulates stomach emptying and signaling to the brain whether the stomach is empty or full. Electrical stimulation blocks nerve activity between the brain and the stomach. By temporarily blocking this nerve traffic, the device reduces the feeling of hunger and enhances the feeling of fullness. The specific mechanisms for weight loss with use of the device are not yet known. In a clinical trial, a little more than half the patients in the experimental group lost at least 9.5 percent of their total weight. We expect this device will be of greatest use along with medical treatments that work in different ways.

**Side Effects:** Pain at the neuroregulator site, vomiting, heartburn, problems swallowing, belching, mild nausea, chest pain.

### INTRAGASTRIC BALLOONS

Intragastric balloons, like Orbera and ReShape, work by taking up space in, and putting pressure on, the inside of the stomach, reducing the amount of food you have to eat to feel full. The balloon is put into the stomach with an endoscope through the mouth and is taken out the same way six months later. It provides a six-month "kick start" to your weight loss and can help you to lose twenty to thirty-five pounds. A recent study demonstrated a 10.5% weight loss when combined with a behavioral modification program versus 5 percent for the program itself, but some people lost significantly more weight that that.

What happens when the balloon is taken out? Weight could be regained, but with a good behavioral program of diet and physical activity, a significant weight loss can be maintained for six months or more. Balloons in development may not require insertion with a scope, but can be swallowed and inflated with air once inside the stomach.

**Side Effects:** Abdominal discomfort, nausea and vomiting, internal bleeding

## THE ASPIREASSIST

This new device, which is not yet approved but is being tested, works by reducing calories absorbed by the body. During the first hour after a meal, the stomach begins breaking down the food and then passes the food to the intestines, where calories are absorbed. The AspireAssist allows patients to remove about 30 percent of the food from the stomach before it reaches the intestine. A tube is placed in the stomach endoscopically through the mouth. The tube connects to a Skin-Port the size of a poker chip on the outside of the abdomen. The Skin-Port has a valve that can be opened or closed to control the flow of stomach contents. After each meal, the patient empties a portion of the stomach contents into the toilet through the tube by connecting a small, handheld device that aspirates 30 percent of what is in the stomach through the Skin-Port. The aspiration process is performed about twenty minutes after finishing a meal and takes ten to twelve minutes.

The A-Tube is placed during a twenty-minute outpatient procedure that is performed under conscious sedation. The A-Tube is inserted through the mouth using an endoscope. A small skin incision is needed to pull the A-Tube through the skin from the stomach. Patients can usually return home within one to two hours and recovery is quick compared to bariatric surgeries. After the skin has healed around the tube, about ten days after the procedure, the Skin-Port is attached to the end of the A-Tube outside the body. This can be done in five minutes in a doctor's office. Once the Skin-Port is installed, the patient can begin aspirating.

In the first U.S. clinical trial, patients lost an average of forty-six pounds in the first year and fifty pounds by the two-year mark. Results appear to be related to compliance with aspiration after each meal. There is a very low risk of serious complications with this device and it should be inexpensive compared to other procedures. The procedure is reversible. The AspireAssist can be removed by means

Larry had bypass surgery in his late fifties. He went from a high of 247 pounds to a low of 202 pounds. Now in his early sixties, he had begun to gain weight and was up to 213 pounds when he came to the Comprehensive Weight Control Center for a consultation. I prescribed metformin and suggested that he start the day with a protein shake. Then life happened. He developed some health issues, which distracted him. If that wasn't enough, Hurricane Sandy hit, severely damaging his home. The disaster threw Larry off course. He stopped taking his postoperative vitamins and medication. By the time he returned to the Center a year later, he had gained back all the weight he had lost after surgery.

He was ready to concentrate on losing weight again. I prescribed Qsymia. Six months later, he returned to say that the medication was not working. He stopped taking the Qsymia and resumed the bupropion, metformin, and vitamins. He knew he had to pay more attention to what he ate and to moving more. Larry started taking short walks after each meal. Following the Change Your Biology Diet, he was eating more protein and fewer carbs. He loved the plan because he could eat large volumes of food. Six months later, he was down to 197 pounds, a fifty-pound loss. Four months after that, he weighed 180 pounds. New tests detected low thyroid, so I added cytomel to his medications. After five months, he was at an all-time low of 169 pounds. He had lost seventy-eight pounds, 31.5 percent of his starting weight, in fifteen months. Most important, Larry had learned a way to eat that would help him stay slim.

of a fifteen-minute procedure performed under conscious sedation. The A-Tube site usually closes naturally on its own.

Aspirating after each meal and learning to chew well are required to make this therapy work. Lifestyle counseling is important to make sure you receive vital nutrients and get the best result. Healthy diet and exercise changes will increase the benefit from the device. In time, with healthier food choices and increased physical activity, the need to aspirate may be reduced to once a day or less.

**Side Effects:** Most common complications have been abdominal discomfort, rash around the port, and constipation/diarrhea.

## GI DYNAMICS ENDOBARRIER

This technology mimics the mechanism and effects of bypass surgery but through a less invasive, reversible procedure. This technology is now being tested and has not been approved. The trial was stopped in the United States because of liver infections, but the device is being used elsewhere in the world. Delivered endoscopically, through the mouth, the EndoBarrier is a flexible, tube-shaped liner that creates a barrier between ingested food and the duodenum/proximal sections of the intestine. The EndoBarrier extends about two feet through the small intestine. Partially digested food passes through the stomach and into the EndoBarrier. The normal action of the intestine moves the food through the EndoBarrier. Bile and enzymes mix together with the food at the end of the EndoBarrier.

The EndoBarrier is not designed to remain in the body permanently. It is being tested in the U.S. for a treatment period of up to twelve months in patients with type 2 diabetes, but can be removed at any time. In clinical trials subjects lost an average of 20 percent of their total body weight within one year and reached healthy blood sugar levels. Initial studies have demonstrated that EndoBarrier therapy's benefits on glycemic control and weight loss have been sustained up to six months and perhaps longer after the device has been removed.

**Side Effects:** Most common complications have been abdominal discomfort, nausea and vomiting, gastrointestinal bleeding, and liver infection.

• • •

Overcoming weight problems can be challenging, but treating weight problems and obesity is becoming more sophisticated every day. If one treatment doesn't work for a patient, we try something else, and the number of options from which we can choose is growing. Though finding the right treatment or combination of treatments can require trial and error, we do not give up. On a practical level, we are helping our patients lose weight successfully. At the same time, on a theoretical level, we are doing scientific research to find the answers that will put a stop to the obesity epidemic. I look forward to the day that all health care providers are educated about how to treat weight problems, so that patients can find help as soon as they start putting on weight, before complications develop.

# AFTERWORD

JUST AS OUR PROGRAM at Weill Cornell Medicine is called the Comprehensive Weight Control Center, my aim in writing this book is to give you a comprehensive understanding of what is going on in your body when you have difficulty maintaining a healthy weight, and the best treatments available for your condition. This is not a typical diet book. It encompasses everything you need to know about weight loss. I backed up the recommendations from our Change Your Biology Plan with hard science, because you need to know why making these changes in your life will help you to lose weight and keep it off. Providing you with an overview of the latest research and new fields of study that are getting closer to finding even more targeted treatments and solutions for this chronic illness should encourage you not to give up and resign yourself to an ever-expanding waistline. Keep trying to control what is in your power to manage—what you eat and how much you move. I believe you will see results if you follow the program. Most people do.

The Quick Start Change Your Biology Diet and the Change Your Biology Diet are meant to be flexible. You have to experiment to see what works well for you. Tailoring your diet to suit your tastes and hunger threshold will make it easier to stay with it. If you stall suddenly and can't make your weight budge below a certain point, change what you are doing. If you have added carbs to your diet, do without them for a while. Try a couple of days on the Quick Start Diet even one day twice per week to jump-start additional weight loss. Add some interval aerobics training to your work out to rev up your metabolism. If you haven't lost 5 percent of your weight after six months on the program or you can't break through a plateau, talk to your doctor or see an obesity medicine specialist. I have provided you with detailed information about the medical and surgical options so you have the background for an informed conversation with your health care providers. Stay determined and keep trying.

The advice you found in these pages is state of the art at this time. As you have seen, breakthroughs and discoveries are happening at lightning speed because so much effort is going into stopping this epidemic illness. I spend a good deal of time reviewing new research, and it's hard to keep up. To stay informed, I suggest you check our website www.cybd.org. The site combines practical advice on diet and exercise, including recipes, menus, exercise tips, and pertinent topics such as how to stay on track when eating out or how to get through the holidays without gaining weight, as well as accessible reports on the latest research findings. You will also be able to order protein shakes and bars that are only available at doctors' offices. Check out the site periodically to keep yourself motivated.

In my efforts to raise awareness in primary care physicians, I have developed an evidence-based weight loss program called BMIQ to which health care professions can subscribe. BMIQ provides the tools and resources needed to implement a weight management program. The program combines office visits with online integrated food, activity, weight and goal tracking tools and program materials, including meal plans and menus. If you need more support, you should mention the program to your doctor. The website is www .BMIQ.com. I want to get the word out to primary care physicians so that they can help their patients at the first sign of a weight problem.

As you lose weight, you will feel so much better. Almost all my patients report a boost in energy and a lift in spirits as weight loss kicks in. They feel lighter in every way. There is nothing like the moment when you notice that your clothing is getting loose. They are proud of what they are accomplishing instead of being down on themselves as they were in the past. Their self-esteem and confidence rise. They become more engaged with everything life has to offer. When I see these transformations, which I am happy to report I do often, it makes me glad to be doing what I do. I wrote this book because so many people had asked me to, urging me to share what we know with more people than we can possibly see at the Comprehensive Weight Control Center. I hope that *The Change Your Biology Diet* will help you reach a healthy weight and stay there, and that you experience the same triumphant joy as so many of our patients do. You have the information you need and a plan to make it happen. Commit yourself to change, and you will succeed.

## ACKNOWLEDGMENTS

EVERY BREAKTHROUGH IN SCIENCE builds on work that has gone on before. I am grateful to my colleagues and collaborators at research centers all over the world who are studying obesity and related metabolic disorders. Their findings inspire our studies. I cite their abundant research in the notes.

At Weill Cornell Medicine, so many outstanding people have supported me in the course of my thirty years of studying obesity, especially Sandy and Joan Weill, who have elevated our entire field through their interest and generosity.

Bill Berkley and Michael Steinhardt have been an invaluable source of wisdom and sage advice.

The Comprehensive Weight Control Center keeps me grounded in the real-life problems of people who are struggling to lose weight. I thank the superb medical and research staff of the Center for their enthusiasm, vision, and sensitivity to the plight of our patients: Our dietitians, Janet L. Feinstein, MS, RD, CDN and Rachel A. Lustgarten, MS, RD, CDN for their many contributions and edits. Dr. Jonathan A. Waitman, Dr. Rekha B. Kumar, Dr. Alpana P. Shukla, Dr. Leon I. Igel, Nurse Practitioner Joy Pape, and Research Coordinator Catherine Thomas.

I want to thank Lupe Minero for her competent development and administration of our BMIQ website.

I thank our entire staff for their compassion, professionalism, and equanimity in a very busy place: Tony Nepomuceno, Arnetia Maddux, Divanessa Bernal, Jade Minto-Johnson, Elisa Barriero, Sandra Lee Colon, and Elizabeth Garcia.

Thanks to David Vigliano, my brilliant literary agent, who found the right publisher for *The Change Your Biology Diet* and introduced me to Diane Reverand many years ago. Diane had been encouraging me to write this book for some time. She was so committed to the project that she ended up being my co-author. She had a vision for the book from the start and has provided valuable insight at every step of the process. Our collaboration has been a pleasure.

Everyone at Houghton Mifflin Harcourt has been passionate about this book. I am so fortunate to be working with Justin Schwartz, Cynthia Brzostowski, Megan Wilson, Natalie Chapman, Lori Glazer, Allison Renzulli, and Marina Padakis Lowry.

Thanks to my wife, Jane, for her invaluable support in helping me to do everything else I'm supposed to do in my life. This book couldn't have happened without her. My mother, Terry, and sister, Adrienne, have provided ample inspiration for me since childhood. Finally, I want to thank my children, Allison and Louis, for being such good kids, and providing comic relief.

SELECTED SOURCES

# Chapter 1

Aronne LJ. Obesity as a Disease: Etiology, Treatment, and Management Considerations for the Obese Patient. *Obesity Research*. 2 December 2002. 10, 2 :95s-96s.

Aronne LJ. Treating Obesity: A New Target for Prevention of Coronary Heart Disease. Prog Cadiovasc Nurs. 2001; 16 (3). http://www .medscape.comeviewarticle/407755_prinyt.

Aronne LJ, Nelinson DS, Lillo JL. Obesity as a Disease State: A New Paradigm for Diagnosis and Treatment. *Clinical Cornerstone*. 9,4: 9-25.

Aronne LJ. Dialogue Box Clincal Cornerstone. 9,4: 26-29.

Bray GA, Clearfield MB, Fintel DJ, Nelinson DS. Overweight and Obesity: The Pathogenesis of Cardiometabolic Risk. *Clinical Cornerstone*. 9, 4: 30-40.

Cannon CP, Kumar A. Treatment of Overweight and Obesity: Lifestyle, Pharmacologic, and Surgical Options. *Clinical Cornerstone*. 9, 4: 55-68.

DeNino WF, Korner J, Aronne LJ. Central control of energy homeostasis. *Current Opinion in Endocrinology & Diabetes*. 2003; 10:330-333.

Igel LI, Powell AG, Apovian, CM, Aronne, LJ. Advances in Medical Therapy for Weight Loss and the Weight Centric Management of Type 2 Diabetes Mellitus. *Curr Atheroscler Rep*. 24 November 2011. Springer. DOU1007/s11883-011-0221-0.

Korner J, Aronne LJ. Obesity. *Integrative Medicine* by Rakel, D. Saunders; 1st edition (June 15, 2002), 257-265.

Korner J, AronneLJ. The emerging science of body weight regulation and its impact on obesity treatment. *The Journal of Clinical Investigation*. March 2003; III, 5: 565-570.

Quan, Martin. Introduction. *Clinical Cornerstone*. 2009; 9,4: 7-8.

Shai I, Jianq R, Manson JE, Willett WC, Colditz GA, HuFB. Ethnicity, obesity and the risk of type 2 diabetes in women: a 20 year follow up study.

Toth PP, Pathophysiology of Obesity: Interplay of Insulin Resistance and Comorbidities. *Obesity Consults*. August 2013; 1, 2: 6-8.

Wang J, Thornton JC, Burastero S, Shen J, Tanenbaum S, Heymsfield SB, Pierson RN. obes Res, July 1996; 4 (4). 377–84.

Wright SM, Aronne LJ. Causes of obesity. *Abdominal Imaging*. October 2012. 37, 5: 730-732.

# Chapter 2

## ON OBESITY DRIVERS:

Keith SW, Et. Al. Putative contributors to the secular increase in obesity: exploring the roads less traveled. *International Journal of Obesity*. (2006) 30, 1585-1594.

Swinburn BA, Sacks G, Hall KD, McPherson K, Finegood DT, Moddie ML, Gortmaker, SL. The global obesity pandemic: shaped by global drivers and local environments. *The Lancet*. August 27,2011; 378: 804-14.

## ON EPIGENETICS:

Adams J. (2008) *Obesity*, epigenetics, and gene regulation. *Nature Education* 9(1):128.

Campion J, Milagro FI, Martinez JA. Individuality and epigenetics in obesity. Journal compilation C 2009 International Association for the study of obesity. Obesity reviews 10, 383-392.

Champion J, Milagro F, Martinez JA. Epigenetics and obesity. *Prog Mol Biol Transl Sci*. 2010;94:291-347. Doi: 10.1016/S1877-1173(10)94011-8.

Eating for your epigenome. http://epigenome.eu/en/2,48,875.

Ellis, Marie. Epigenetic mechanism found that could tackle obesity's effects. *Medical News Today*. MediLexicon, Intl. 13 March 2014. Web. 15 Oct 2014. http://www.medical newstoday.com /articles/273881.php.

Franks PW, Ling C. Epigenetics and obesity: the devil is in the details. *BMC Medicine*. 2010, 8:88. Doi:10.1186/1741-7015-8-88.

Haggard P, Nutrition and the epigenome.*Prog Mol Biol Transl Sci*. 2012; 108:427-46 doi:10.1016/B978-0-12-398397-8.00016-2.

Herrera BM, Keildson, S, LIndgre CM. Genetics and epigenetics of obesity. *Maturitas*. May 2011; 69(1):41-48. Doi: 10.1016/j. maturitas.2011.02.018.

Martinez, JA. Body-weight regulation: causes of obesity. Proceedings of the Nutrition Society August 2000; 59(3):337-345. http:// journals.cambridge.org/action/displayAbstract?frompage= online&aid+797112fileld=S0029665100000380.

Milagro FI, Mansego ML, DeMiguel C, Martinez JA. Dietary factors, epigenetic modifications and obesity outcomes: progresses and perspectives. *Mol Aspects Med*. 2013 Jul-Aug; 34(4): 7892-812. Doi: 10.1016/j.mam.2012.06.010. Epub 2012 Jul 4.

Parker-Pope T. Lost Sleep Can Lead to Weight Gain. *New York Times*. March 18, 2013. http://well.blogs.nytimes.com/2013/03/18/ lost-sleep-can-lead-to-weight-gain/.

Nutrition and the Epigenome. http://learn.genetics.utah.edu/content /epigenetics/nutrition/.

Ronn T, Et. Al. 2013. A six months exercise intervention influences the genome wide DNA methylation pattern in human adipose tissue. PLOS Genetics 9(6): e1003572. Doi:10.1371/journal.pgen.1003572.

Samani NJ, Et. Al. DNA methylation and body-mass index: a genome wide analysis. *The Lancet*. Published online 13 March 2014. DOI: http://dx.doi.org10.1016/s0140-6736 (13) 62674-4.

Seki Y, Williams L, Vuguin PM, Charron MJ. 2012. Minireviews: Epigenetic programming of diabetes and obesity: animal models. *Endocrinology* 153:1032-1038.

Stoger R. Epigenetics and obesity. *Pharmacogenomics*. Dec 2008: 9 (12): 1851-1860. Doi: 10.2217/14622416.9.121851.

Youngson NA, Morris MJ. What obesity research tells us about epigenetic mechanisms. *Phil. Trans, R. Soc. B* 2013 368, 20110337, publishing 19 November 2012.


ON SLEEP DEPRIVATION

Benedict C, Et. Al. Acute sleep deprivation enhances the brain's response to hedonic food stimuli: an fMRI study. *J Clin Endocrinol Metab.* 2012 Mar; 97 (3):E443-7) doi: 10.1210/jc.2011-2759. E pub 2012 Jan 18.

Donga E, Et. Al.. A single night of partial sleep deprivation induces insulin resistance in multiple metabolic pathways in healthy subjects. *J Clin Endocrinol Metab.* 2010 Jun;95(6):2983-8. Doi:1210/jc:2009 -2430. Epub 2010 Apr 6.

Gardner, A. Too little sleep may fuel insulin resistance. Health.com. October 16, 2012. http://www.cnn.com/2012/10/15/health/sleep -insulin-resistance/index.html.

Harmon, Katherine. How slight sleep deprivation could add extra pounds. *Scientific American*. Oct. 24, 2012. http://www.scientific american.com/article/sleep-deprivation-obesity/?print=true.

O'Connor A. How sleep loss adds to weight gain. *New York Times*. August 6, 2013. http://well.blogs.nytimes.com/2013/08/06/ how-sleep-loss-adds-to-weight-gain/?_php+true&_type+blogs&_r+0.

Parker-Pope T. Lost sleep can lead to weight gain. *New York Times*. March 18, 2013. http://well.blogs.nytimes.com/2013/03/18/ lost-sleep-can-lead-to-weight-gain/?_r=0.

Patel SR, HU FB. Short sleep duration and weight gain: a systematic review. *Obesity (Silver Spring)*. 2008; 16:643-53.

Patel SR, Malhotra A, White DP, Gottlieb DJ, Hu FB. Association between reduced sleep and weight gain in women. *Am J Epidemiol.* 2006; 165: 947-54.

Taheri S, Lin L, Austin D, Young T, Mignot E. Short sleep duration is associated with reduced leptin, elevated ghrelin, and increased body mass index. DOI: 0.1371/journl.pmed.0010062.

## DRUGS

Can prescription drugs cause weight gain? http://www.drugs.com/article/weight-gain.html.

Kyle T, Kuehl B. Prescription medications and weight gain—what you need to know. http://www.obesityaction.org/educational -resources/resoourcearticles-2/general -articles/prescription -medications-weight-gain.

Laino D. Is your medicine cabinet making you fat? http://www.webmd .com/a-to-z-guides/features/is-your-medicine-cabinet-making-you-fat.

## AMBIENT TEMPERATURE

Cell Press. Exposure to cold temperatures can help boost weight loss. Science Daily. Science Daily, 22 January 2013. www.sciencedaily .com/releases/2014/01/140122133824.htm].

Ellis M. "Good" brown fat stimulated by cold , study shows. http:// www.medicalnewstoday.com/articles/278646.php.

Garvan Institute of Medical Research. Embrace the cold: Evidence that shivering and exercise may convert white fat to brown. Feb. 4, 2014. http://www.sciencedaily.com/releases/2014/02/140204123619.htm.

Lee, P, Et. Al. Temperature-acclimated brown adipose tissue modulates insulin sensitivity in humans. *Diabetes,* doi: 10.2337/db14-0513, published online 22 June 2014, Abstract.

To what degree is a person's body weight affected by the ambient temperature and humidity? Do we conserve or release water as the climate changes? *Scientific American.* June 11, 2007. http://www.scientific american.com/article/experts-body-weight-ambient-temperature/.

van Marken Lichtenbelt W, Kingma B, van der Lans A, and Schellen L. Cold Exposure—an approach to increasing energy expenditure in humans. Cell Press. *Trends in Endocrinology & Metabolism,* January 2014.


## ENDOCRINE DISRUPTORS

Ahearn A. What do we know about obesogens? With Bruce Blumberg (podcast) *Environ Health Perspect* 120 (2012); http://dx.doi .org/10.1289/ehp.trp070212 (Online 2 July 2012).

Environmental Working Group. Dirty Doze List of Endocrine Disruptors. October 28, 2013. http://www.ewg.org/research/ dirty-doze-list-endocrine-disruptors.

Garcia-Arevalo M, Et. Al. Exposure to bisphenal-A during pregnancy partially mimics the effects of a high-fat diet altering glucose homeostasis and gene expression in adult male mice. *Plos One.* 2014 June 24; 9(6):e100214. Doi: 10.1371/journal.pone.0100214. eCollection.

Grun F, Blumberg B. Minireview: the case for obesogens. *Mol Endocrinol.* Aug 2009; 23 (8): 1127-1134.

Heindel, JJ. Endocrine Disruptors and the Obesity Epidemic. *Toxicological Sciences* 76, 247-249 (2003) doi: 10.1093/toxsci /kfg255.

Karoutsou E, Polymeris A. Environmental endocrine disruptors and obesity. *Endo Regul.* 2012 Jan; 46(1):37-46.

Kristof, Nicholas D. Warnings from a flabby mouse. *New York Times.* Jan. 19, 2013. http://www.nytimes.com/2013/01/20/opinion/sunday /kristof-warnings-from-a-flabby-mouse.html?_r+0.

National Institute of Environmental Health Sciences. Endocrine Disruptors. May 2010. www.niehs.nih.gov.

Newbald RR, Padila-Banks E, Jefferson WN, Heindel JJ. Effects of endocrine disruptors on obesity. *Int J Androl.* 2008 Apr; 31 (2): 201-208. Doi:10.1111/j.1365-2605.2007.00858.x.

Newbold RR. Impact of environmental endocrine disrupting chemicals on the development of obesity. *Hormones* 2010, 9(3):206-217/.

What are endocrine disruptors? http://www.epa.gov/endo/pubs /edspovervieew/whatare.htm.

## SOCIAL NETWORK

Christakis NA, Fowler JH. The Spread of Obesity in a Large Social Network over 32 years. *N Engl j med* 2007; 357:370-379. July 26, 2007. Doi:10.1056/NEJMa066082.

Cohen-Cole E, Fletcher JM. Is obesity contagious? Social networks vs. environmental factors in the obesity epidemic. *Journal of Health Economics*. 2008: (27) 5: 1382-1387.

Harmon K. How obesity spreads in social networks. *Scientific American*. May 5, 2011. http://www.cientificamerican.com/article /social-spread-obesity/.

Komaroff A. Social networks can affect weight, happiness. Dec.16, 2011. http://www.health.harvard.edu/blog/social -networks-can-affect-weight-happiness-201112163983.

Thompson, Clive. Are your friends making you fat? *New York Times*. Sept. 13, 2009. http://www.nytimes.com/2009/09/13.magazine /13contagion-t.html?pagewanted=print.

## ADENOVIRUS

Atkinson RL, Dhurandhar NV, Allison DB, Bowen, RL, Israel BA, Albu JB, Augustus AS. 2005 Human adenovirus-36 is associated with increased body weight and paradoxical reduction of serum limps. *Int. J.Obesity* 29:281-286.

Atkinson, RL. Virus-induced obesity in humans. http://microbemaga-zine.org/index.php?option+com_content&view=article&id=5068: virus-induced-obesity-in -humans&itemid+1251.

Cimons, M. Can an upper-respiratory infection make you fat? If it's cause by adenovirus 36, maybe. *Washington Post*. December 9, 2013. http://www.washingtonpost.com/national/health-science/ dab-an-upper-respiratory-infection-make-you-fat-if-its-caused-by

-adenovirus 36, maybe /2013/12/06/8104772c-4895-11
e3-a196-3544a03c2351_story.html.

Durandhar NV. Is obesity caused by an adenovirus. *Expert Rev
Anti Infect Ther.* 2012; 10(5):521-524. Oct. 3, 2012. http://
blogs.plos.org/obsitypanacea/2012/10/03/infectobesity-is
-transmitted-thrugh-a-common-viral-infection/.

Saunders T. Infectobesity: is obesity transmitted through a common viral
infection?.

# Chapter 3

Berthoud, HR. The vagus nerve, food intake and obesity. Regul Pept.
August 7, 2008.149 (1-3): 15-25. Published online Mar 25.2008. doi:
10.1016/jregpep.2007.08.024.

Blaut M. Gut microbiota and energy balance: role in obesity, *Proc Nutr
Soc.* 2014 Dec 18: 1-8. (Epub ahead of print).

Cardinelli CS, Sala PC, Alves CC, Torrinhas RS, Waitzberg DL.
Influence of intestinal microbiota on body weight gain: a narrative
review of the literature. *Obes surg.* 2014 Dec 17. (Epub ahead of
print).

Chambers ES, et.al. Effects of targeted delivery of propionate to the human colon on appetite regulation, body weight maintenance, and ad-
iposity in overweight adults. 2014 Dec 10. pii: gutjnl-2014-307913
*Gut/* doi:10.1136/gutjnl-20140397913.

Cox LM, Blaser MJ. Antibiotics in early life and obesity. *Nat rev endocrinol.* 2014 Dec 9.doi: 10.1038/nrendo.2014,210 (Epub ahead of
print).

Delzenne NM, Cani PD, Neyrinck. Modulation of glucagon-like peptide
1 and energy metabolism by inulin and oligofructose: experimental
data. *J Nutr.* 2007 Nov; 137 (11 Supp) 2547S-2551S.

Feehley T, Nagler CR. Health: The weighty costs of non-caloric sweeteners. *Nature.* Volume: 514, Pages: 176–177 Date published: (09
October 2014) DOI: doi:10.1038/nature13752.

Greenhill C. Not so sweet—artificial sweeteners can cause glucose intolerance by affecting the gut microbiota. Journal name: Nature Reviews Endocrinology. Volume: 10, Page: 637 Year published: (2014). DOI: doi:10.1038/nrendo.2014.167.

Gunnars, K. Why extra virgin olive oil is the healthiest fat on earth. http://authoritynutrition.com/extra-virgin-olive-oil/.

Haiken, M. The new theory on weight loss: your bad diet has damaged your brain. http://www.forbes.com/sites/melaniehaiken/2013/08/21 /the-real-secret-to-losing-weight-from-a-top-expert/.

Health benefits of the Mediterranean diet. http://www.ppatient.co.uk /print9221.

Inui A. Feeding and body-weight regulation by hypothalamic neuropeptides—mediation of the actions of leptin. *Trends Neurosci.* 1999 Feb; 22(2):62-7.

Innes, Emma. Could olive oil be the key to weight loss? Scientists discover even the smell of it can make us feel full. *Daily Mail.* 15 March 2013. http://www.dailymail.co.uk/health/article-2293948/Could-olive-oil-key-weight-loss-Scientists-discover-SMELL-make-feel -full.html.

Kral JG, Paez W, Wolfe BM. Vagal nerve function in obesity: therapeutic implications. *World J Surg.* 2009 Oct. 33(10) a995-2006. Doi: 10:1007/s00268-009-0138-8.

Kyle T, Hignett W. Ghrelin the "go" hormone. http://www.obesityaction.org/educational-resources/resource-articles-2/general-articles /ghrelin-the-go-hormone.

Maki KC, Phillips AK. Dietary substitutes for refined carbohydrate that show promise for reducing risk of type 1 diabetes in men and women. *J nutr.* 2015 Jan; 145 (1):159S-63S. doi: 10,3945/ jn.114.195149. Epub 2014 Dec 3.

Marshall JA, Bessesen DH. Dietary Fat and the Development of Type 2 *Diabetes. Diabetes Care/* March 2002. 25 (3):620-622. Doi: 1-.2337 /diacare.25.3.620.

Martin-Pelaez S, Covas MI, Fito M, Kusar A, Pravst I. Health effects of olive oil polyphenols: recent advances and possibilities for the use of health claims. *Mol Nutr Food Res.* 2012 May; 57 (5):760-71. Doi: 10.1002/mnfr.201200421. Epub 2013 Mar 1.

McNay DE, Speakman JR. High fat diet causes rebound weight gain. *Mol Metab.* 2012 Nov 2; 2(2):103-8. Doi: 10.1016/j/molmet.2012.10.003.eCollection 2012.

Musilova S, Et. Al. Prebiotic effects of a novel combination of galactooligosaccharides and maltodextrins. *J Med Food.* 2014 Dec 19. (epub ahead of print).

Obesity damages vagal nerves. *Bariatric News.* http://www.bariatric news.net/?q=print/news/111162/obesity-damages-vagal-nerves.

Olive oil, extra virgin. http://www.whfoods.com/genpage.php?tname =foodspice&dbid=132.

Perez-Jimenez F, Et. Al. International conference on the healthy effect of virgin olive oil. *Eur J Clin Invest* 2005 Jul; 35 (7) 421-4.

Perry, B, Wang, Y. Appetite regulation and weight control: the role of gut hormones. *Nutrition and Diabetes* (2012) 2, e26; http://www.nature.com/nutdjournal/v2/n1/full/nutd201121a.html.doi:10.1038/nutd.2011.21.

Rohner-Jeanrenaud F, Hochstrasser AC, Jenrenaud B. Hyperinsulinemia of preobese and obese fa/fa/ rats is partly vagus nerve mediated. Am J Physiol. 1983 Apr; 244(4):E317-22.

Ryssdal, K. Processed foods make up 70 percent of the U.S. diet. March 12, 2013. http://www.marketplace.org/topics/life/big-book /processed-foods-make-70-percent-us-diet.

Shekhar C. Nervy approach to fighting fat. *Los Angeles Times.* http:// articles.latimes.com/print/2008/jun/09/health/he-implant9.

Simpson KA, Martin NM, Bloom SR. Hypothalamic regulation of appetite. Expert rev endocrinol metab. 2008; 3(5):577-592.

Suez J, Et. Al. Artificial sweeteners induce glucose intolerance by altering the gut microbiota. *Nature.* 2014 Oct 9; 514 (7521): 181-6. Doi: 10.1038/nature 13793. Epub 2014 Sep 17.

Yon MA, Mauger SL, Pickavance LC. Relationship between dietary macronutrients and adult neurogenesis in the regulation of energy metabolism. *British Journal of Nutrition* (2013) 109: 1573-1589.

Xu, H Et. Al. Chronic inflammation in fat plays a crucial role in the development of obesity-elated insulin resistance. *J Clin Invest.* 2003; 112 (12): 1821-1830. Coi:10.1172/JCI119451.

# Chapter 4

Added Sugars. http://www.heart.org/HEARTORG/Getting healthy /NutritionCenter/HealthyDietGoals/Sugars-and-Carbohydrates _UCM_303296_Article.jsp%20.

*Ann Intern Med.* 2014;161(5):309-318. doi:10.7326/M14-0180

Astrup A, Raben A, Geiker N. The role of higher protein diets in weight control and obesity-related comorbidities. *Int J Obes* (London) 20145 Dec 26. Doi: 10.1038/ijo.2014.216. (Epub ahead of print).

Bazzano, LA, Et. Al. Effects of Low-Carbohydrate and Low-Fat Diets: A Randomized Trial.

Blackshaw S, Lee DA, Et. Al.. Tanycytes of the hypothalamic median eminence form a diet-responsive neurogenenic niche. *Nat Neurosci.* 2012 March 25; 15 (5): 700-02. Published online 2012 Mr 25. Doi: 10.1038/nn.3079.

Bosse JD, Dixon, BM. Dietary protein in weight management: a re-view proposing protein spread and change theories. *Nutrition and Metabolism.* 2012. 9:81. http://www.nutrition andmetabolism.com /content/9/1/81. Doi:10.1186/1743-7075-9-81/.

Carbohydrates. http://www.cdc.gov/nutrition/everyone/basics/carbs.html.

Carbohydrates and health: Not that simple...or that complex. http://www .health.harvard.edu/newsweek/Carbohydratews-and-Health.htm.

Chen M, Et. Al. Dairy consumption and risk of type 2 diabetes: 3 co-horts of US adults and an updated meta-analysis. *BMC Medicine* 2014, 12: 215 doi:10.1186/s12916-014-0215-1.

Diabetolgia. Study shows yogurt consumption reduces the risk of type 2 diabetes. Science Daily, 5 February 2014. http://www.sciencedaily .com/releases/2014/02/140205184736.htm.

DiNicolantonio JJ, Lucan SC. Sugar Season. It's Everywhere, and Addictive. *New York Times.* The Opinion Pages. Dec 22, 2014.

Donahoo W, Et. Al. Dietary fat increases energy intake across the range of typical consumption in the United States. *Obesity* (Silver Spring) 20008 Jan; 16 (1): 64-9. Doi: 10.1038/ooby.2007.31.

Feinman RD, Pogozelski W, et.al. Dietary carbohydrate restriction as the first approach in diabetes management critical review and evidence base. *The Journal of Nutrition.* January 2015. 31 (1): 1-13. Doi: http://dx.doi.org/10.1016/jnut.2014.06.011.

Foster-Powell K, Holt SHA, Brand-Miller JC. International table of glycemic index and glycemic load values. *American Journal of Clinical Nutrition.* 20021,2. http://acjn.nutrition.org/content26/1/5.fullpdf.

Fructose vs. glucose. http://www.diffen.com/difference/Fructose _vs_Glucose.

Fructose vs glucose: what's worse? http://www.precisionnutrition.com /research-review-fructuse-vs-glucose.

Glycemic index and glycemic load for 100+ foods. http://www .health.harvard.edu/healthy-eating/glycemic_index_and -glycemic_load_for_100_foods.

Gunnars, K. Daily intake of sugar—how much sugar should you eat per day? http://authoritynutrition.com/how-much-sugar-per-day.

Harvie, M, Et. Al. The effect of intermittent energy and carbohydrate restriction v. daily energy restriction on weight loss and metabolic disease risk markers in overweight women. *British Journal of Nutrition* (2013) 110, 1534-1547. doi: 1017/S00071145130000792.

Larsen, TM, Et. Al. (2010). Diets with high or low protein content and glycemic index for weight-loss maintenance. *New England Journal of Medicine,* 363, 2101-13.

Leidy, HJ, Et. Al. (2007) Higher protein intake preserves lean mass and satiety with weight loss in pre-obese and obese women. *Obesity,* 15 (2): 421-29.

Lejeune MPG, Kovaks EMR, Westerterp-Plantega MS. (2005) Additional protein intake limits weight regain after weight loss in humans. *British Journal of Nutrition,* 93: 281-89.

Lima, C. The 57 names of sugar. http://www.prevention.com/print /39336.

Neurogenesis spurred by a high-fat diet encourages more eating and fat storage, animal study suggests. May 21, 2012. http://www.hopkinsmedicine.org/news/media/releases/ weight_struggles_blame_new_neurons_in_your_hypothalamus.

O'Connor LM, Et. Al. Dietary dairy product intake and incident type 2 diabetes: a prospective study using dietary data from a 7-day food diar. *Diabetologia*, 22014. Doi: 10.1007/s00125 -014-3176-1.

Page KA, Et. Al. Effects of fructose vs. glucose on regional cerebral blood flow in brain regions involved with appetite and reward pathways. *JAMA*. 2013 Jan2; 309(1):63-30. Doi: 10.1001/ jama.2012.116975.

Simple vs. complex carbs. http://www.diabetes.co.uk/nutrition/simple -carbs-vs-complex-carbs.html.

Stanhope KL, Havel PJ. Endocrine and metabolic effects of consuming beverages sweetened with fructose, glucose, sucrose, or high fructose corn syrup. *Am J Clin Nutr.* 2008 Dec. 88(6):1733S-1737S. doi: 10.3945/ajcn.2008.258225D.

Stanhope KL, Havel PJ. Fructose consumption: recent results and their potential implications. *Ann N Y Academy Sci.* 2010 Mar:1190:15 -24. Doi 10.111j/1749-6632.2009.05266.x.

Weigle DS, Et. Al. A high-protein diet induces sustained reductions in appetite, ad libitum caloric intake, and body weight despite compensatory changes in diurnal plasma leptin and ghrelin concentrations 1'2'3. *Am J Clin Nutr.* July 2005 82 (1): 41-48.

# Chapter 5

Amandine C, Zarrinpar A, Panda S. Time-restricted feeding is a preventative and therapeutic intervention against diverse nutritional challenges. *Cell Metabolism*. December 2, 2014. 20, 991-1005.

Fetters KA. The Secret Ingredient for weight loss: does your breakfast have enough of it? November 15, 2013. http://www.womenshealth mag.com/weight-loss/high-protein-breakfast.

Gray BB. Saving Carbs for Dinnertime Might Help Control Weight.

Dec. 13, 2012. *U.S. News.* http://news.health.com/2012/12/14/
saving-carbs-for-dinnertime-might-help-control-weight/.

Pellegrini A. High-protein breakfast & weight loss. Jan. 14, 2014. http://
livestrong.com/article/280195-high-protein-breakfast-weight-loss/.

Sofer S, Et. Al. Greater weight loss and hormonal changes after 6 months diet with carbohydrates eating mostly at dinner.
*Obesity (Silver Spring).* 2011 Oct; 19 (10):2006-14. Doi: 10.1038/
oby.2011.48. (Epub 2011 Apr).

Turner N. The best time to eat for weight loss. April 18, 2012. *Women's
Health Magazine.* http://www.womenshealthmag.com/weight-loss
/best-time-to-eat.

# Chapter 6

Ashley J, St. Jeor S, Perumean-Chaney S, Schrage J, and Bovee V. Meal
Replacements in Weight Intervention. Obesity Research. 2001; 9:
312S-320S.

Cheskin L, Mitchell A, Jhaveri A, Mitola A, Davis L, Lewis R, Yep M,
and Lycan M. Efficacy of Meal Replacements Versus a Standard
Food-Based Diet for Weight Loss in Type 2 Diabetes: A Controlled
Clinical Trial. The Diabetes Educator. 2008; 34: 118-127.

Davis LM, et al. Efficacy of a meal replacement diet plan compared to a
food-based diet plan after a period of weight loss and weight maintenance: a randomized controlled trial. *Nutrition Journal* 2010; 9:11.

Ditschunett H, Flechtner-Mors M. Value of Structured Meals for Weight
Management: Risk Factors and Long-Term Weight Maintenance.
Obesity Research. 2001; 9: 284S-289S.

Fletchtner-Mors M, Et. Al. Enhanced weight loss with protein–enriched
meal replacements in subjects with the metabolic syndrome. *Diabetes
Metab Res Rev.* 2010 Jul; 26(5):393-405. Doi: 10.1002/dmrr.1097.

Heymsfield SR. "Meal replacements and energy balance." Physiology
and Behavior. 2010; 100: 90-94.

Heymsfield SB, van Mierlo CAJ, van der Knapp HCM, Heo M, and
Frier HI. Weight Management Using a Meal Replacement Strategy:

Meta and Pooling Analysis from Six Studies. International Journal of Obesity. 2003; 27: 537-549.

Konig D, Deibert P, Frey I, Landmann U, Berg A. Effect of Meal Replacement on Metabolic Risk Factors in Overweight and Obese Subjects. Annals of *Nutrition and Metabolism*. 2008; 52:74-78.

Noakes M, Foster P, Keogh J, and Clifton P. Meal Replacements are as Effective as Structured Weight-Loss Diets for Treating Obesity in Adults with Features of Metabolic Syndrome. *The Journal of Nutrition*. 2004; 134: 1894-1899.

Rohrer JE, Takahashi P. Should overweight and obese primary care patients be offered a meal replacement diet? *Obesity Research and Clinical Practice*. 2008; 2:263-268.

Seagle H, Strain GW, Makris A, and Reeves R. Position of the American Dietetic Association: Weight Management. Journal of the American Dietetic Association. 2009; 109: 330-346.

Taylor MG. Choosing a protein powder. http://www.nutrition expresss.com/article+index/authors/mark+g+taylor+ms/.show article.aspx?articleid=896.

# Chapters 7 and 8

The Change Your Biology Diet material is based on the information we give our patients at the Weill Cornell Center for Weight Control as well as material from the website BMIQ, an online, comprehensive weight loss program developed for health care professionals at https://www.bmiq.com/.

# Chapter 9

The recipes were inspired and adapted from magazines, cookbooks, and websites. There are many fine websites where you can find healthy recipes that are caloric bargains. For example:

http://www.health.com
http://www.eatingwell.com

www.cookinglight.com
www.myrecipes.com
www.allrecipes.com
www.foodnetwork.com
www.marthastewart.com
www.skinnytaste.com

# Chapter 10

Sitting disease" by the numbers. http://www.juststand.org/tabid/674/language/en-us/default.aspx.

Adamson S, Et. Al. High intensity training improves health and physical function in middle-aged adults. *Biology*. 2014, 3, 333-344. Doi: 10.3390/biology302333.

Bruno NE, Et. Al. Creb coactivators direct anabolic responses and enhance performance of skeletal muscle. EMBO J. 2014 May 2; 33(9): 1027-43. doi: 10.1002/embj.201386145. Epub 2014 Mar 27.

Calorie burner: How much better is standing up than sitting? 16 October 2013. *BBC News Magazine*. http://www.bbc.com/news/magazome-24532996?print+true.

Dunstan DW, Et. Al. High-intensity resistance training improves glycemic control in older patients with type 2 diabetes. *Diabetes Care*. October 2002. 25(10):1729-36.

Francois ME, Et. Al. "Exercise snacks" before meals: a novel strategy to improve glycaemic control in individuals with insulin resistance . *Diabetologia*, 2o143.doi: 10.1007/s00125-014-3244-6.

Gillen JB, Et. Al. Three minutes of all-out intermittent exercise per week increases skeletal muscle oxidative capacity and improves cardiometabolic health. Nov. 3, 2014 *Plos One* 9(11): e111489. Doi:10.1371/journal.pone.0111489.

Hagerman FC, Et. Al. Effects of high-intensity resistance training on untrained older men: strength, cardiovascular, and metabolic responses. *J gerontol A boil Sci Med Sci* (2000) 55 (7): B336-B346. Doi: 10.1093/Gerona/55.7.B336.

Hamilton MT, Hamilton DG, Zderic TW. Role of low energy

expenditure and sitting in Obesity, metabolic syndrome, type 2 diabetes, and cardiovascular disease. *Diabetes.* Nov 2007. 56: 2655-67.

Klein S. An unexpected exercise that targets belly fat. *Huffington Post.* Dec 22, 2014. http://www.huffingtonpost.com/2014/12/22/weight -lifting-belly-fat_n_6367756.html.

Kolata G. Brown Fat, Triggered by cold or exercise, may yield a key to weight control. January 24, 2012. *New York Times.* http://www .nytimes.com/2012/01/25/health/brown-fat-burns-ordinary-fat-study-finds.html?_r=0&pagewanted=print.

Mischel NA1, Llewellyn-Smith IJ, Mueller PJ. Physical (in)activity-dependent structural plasticity in bulbospinal catecholaminergic neurons of rat rostral ventrolateral medulla. J Comp Neurol. 2014 Feb 15;522(3):499-513. doi: 10.1002/cne.23464.

Nordquist C Stand up for three hours in the office and lose weight. http://www.medicalnewstoday.com/articles/254894.

Ouellet V, Carpentier, AC, Et. Al. Brown adipose tissue oxidative metabolism contributes to energy expenditure during acute cold exposure in humans. *J Clin Invest.* 2012;122(2):545–552. doi:10.1172 /JCI60433.

Reynolds G. How inactivity changes the brain. Jan. 22, 2014. *New York Times,* http://well.blogs.nytimes.com/2014/01/22/how -inactivity-changes-the-brain.

Reynolds G. The scientific 7-minute workout. Oct. 24, 2014. http://well .blogs.nytimes.com/2013/05/09/the-scientific-7-minute-workout/.

Reynolds G. For fitness, push yourself. June 25, 2014. *New York Times.* http://well.blogs.nytimes.com/2014/06/25/for-fitness-push-yourself/.

Reynolds G. The super-short workout and other fitness trends. Dec 31, 2014. *New York Times.* http://well.blogs.nytimes.com/2014/12/31/ the-super-short-workout-and-other-fitness-trends/.

Sjogren P, Fisher R, Kallings L, Svenson U, Roos G, Hellenius M. Stand up for health—avoiding sedentary behavior might lengthen your telomeres: secondary outcomes from a physical activity RCT in older people. *British Journal of Sports Medicine.* Doi: 10.1136/ bjs-2-13-093342.

Tetnowski J. 25 June 2014. *Consumer's Research*. http://consumers research.org/no-pain-no-gain-intense-exercise-may-be-better-for-you.

Vlahos J. Is sitting a lethal activity? April 14, 2011. *New York Times*. http://www.nytimes.com/2011/04/17/magazine/mag-17sitting-t .html?pagewanted=print.

Wang Y, Vera L, Fischer WH, Montminy M. The CREB coactivator CRTC2 links hepatic ER stress and fasting gluconeogenesis. *Nature* 460 534-537 (23 July 2009) doi:10:1038/nature08111.

Watson S, Too much sitting linked to an earl death. *Harvard Health Publications*. http://www.health.harvard.edu/blog/ too-much-sitting-linked-to-an-early-death-201401297004.

Zickerman A, Schley B. *The Power of 10: The Once a Week Slow Motion Fitness Revolution*. New York. HarperCollins Publishers, 2002.

# Chapter 11

Apovian CM, Aronne LJ, Bessesen DH et al., Pharmacological Management of Obesity: An Endocrine Society Clinical Practice Guideline, Feb. 2015, Clin Endocrinol Metab 100(2):342-3612. doi: 10.1210/jc.2014-3415.

Aronne LJ, Et. Al. Evaluation of phentermine and topiramate versus phentermine/topiramate extended-release in obese adults. *Obesity (Silver Spring)*. 2013 Nov; 21(11):2163-71. Doi:10.1002/oby.20584.

Ryan DH. New medications and new ways to use them. Obesity con-sults-med-review 1-36.

Koven S. Diet Drugs Work: Why Won't Doctors Prescribe Them? *New Yorker*. December 4, 2013. http://www.newyorker.com/tech /elements/diet-drugs-work-why-wont-doctors-prescribe-them.

FDA approves weight-management drug Saxenda. FDA News Release. Dec. 23, 2014. http://www.fda.gov/NewsEvents/Newsroom/Press announcements/ucm427913.htm/.

Fujioka K, Ryan DH. Safety and tolerability of medications approved for chronic weight management. Obesity consults-meds-review.

FDA approves weight-management drug Contrave. FDA News Release. Sept. 10, 2014. http://www.fda.gov/NewsEvents/Newsroom/Press Announcements/ucm413896.htm.

Musil R, Obermeier M, Russ P, Hamerle M. Weight gain and antipsychotics: a drug safety review. Expert Opin Drug Saf. 2014 Nov 15: 1-14.

Powell AG, Apovian CM, Aronne LJ. New drug targets for the treatment of obesity. *Nature*. July 2011. 90 (1): 40-51. Doi:10.1038/clpt.2011,82.

# Chapter 12

Apovian CM, Sharaiha P Kedia, N, Kumta,N, DeFilippis, EM, Gaidhane M, Shukla A, Aronne AJ, Kahaleh, MK. Initial experience with endoscopic sleeve gastroplast technical success and reproducibility in the bariatric population. *Endoscopy*. 2015 Feb; 100(2): 342-362. DOI y: http://dx.doi.org/10.1055/s-0034-1390773. Published online: 2014.

Abu Dayyeh BK, Rajan E, Gostout CJ. Endoscopic sleeve gastroplassty: a potential endoscopic alternative to surgical sleeve gastrectomy for treatment of obesity. *Gastrointest Endosc*. 2013 Sep; 78(3):530-5. Doi: 10.1016/j.gie.2013.04.197.

Bariatric surgery procedures. Society for Metabolic and Bariatric Surgery. http://asmbs.org/patients/bariatric-surgery-procedures.

FDA approves first-of-kind device to treat obesity. January 14, 2015. http://www.fda.gov/NewsEvents/Newsroom/PressAnnouncements /ucm430223.htm.

Gaglini S. A sleeve for your small intestine: inteview with GI dynamics founder, Andy Levine.April 10. 2013. http://medgadget.com/2013/04 /a-sleeve-for-your-small-intestine-with-gi-dynamics-founder-andy -levine.html.

Haspel T. Before you conclude that you're gluten-sensitive, consider FODMAPS foods. *Washington Post*. http://www.washingtonpost .com/national/health-science/before-you-conclude-that-youre -gluten-sensitive-consider-fodmaps-foods/2015/02/09/a66349fa- 6c19-11e4-a31c-77759fc1eacc_story.html.

Life after weight-loss surgery. http://www.nlm.nih.gov/medlineplus
/encyc/patientinstructions/000350.htm.

Munzberg H, Laque A, Yu S, Rezai-Zadeh K, Berthoud HR. Appetite
and body weight regulation after bariatric surgery. *Obes Rev.* 2015
Feb; 16 Suppl 1:77-90. Doi:10.111/obr.12258.

Stegemann L. Choosing the "right" wieght-loss surgery procedure. http://www.obesityaction.org/educational-resources/
resource-articles-2/weight-loss-surgery.

Sullivan S1, Et. Al. Aspiration therapy leads to weight loss in obese subjects: a pilot study. Gastroenterology. 2013 Dec;145(6):1245-52
.e1-5. doi: 10.1053/j.gastro.2013.08.056. Epub 2013 Sep 6. http://
www.ncbi.nlm.nih.gov/pubmed/24012983.

Tam CS, Et. Al. Could the 4 mechanisms of bariatric surgery
hold the key for novel therapies? Report from a Pennington
Scientif Symposium. *Ob Rev.* 2011 Nov; 12(11)984-94. Doi:
10.111/j/1467-789X.2011.009902.x.

# Weill Cornell Comprehensive Weight Control Center

The mission of the Comprehensive Weight Control Center at Weill Cornell Medical College is to provide clinical care of the highest standard to address weight gain and metabolic syndrome and to advance understanding of obesity as a disease through clinical research and provider training.

## OUR PHYSICIANS

Louis J. Aronne, MD
Jonathan A. Waitman, MD
Rekha B. Kumar, MD, MS
Leon Igel, MD
Joy Pope, NP

## CONTACT

1165 York Avenue
New York, NY 10065

Phone:
646-962-2111

Fax:
646-962-0159

# ABOUT THE AUTHOR

Louis J. Aronne, MD, FACP, is a leading authority on obesity and its treatment. He is the Sanford I. Weill Professor of Metabolic Research at Weill Cornell Medical College and directs the Comprehensive Weight Control Center and Metabolic Clinical Research, a state-of-the-art, multidisciplinary obesity research and treatment program. He has an adjunct appointment at Columbia University College of Physicians and Surgeons. Dr. Aronne is founder and CEO of BMIQ, a weight control program that is delivered by health care providers to their patients during office visits.

Dr. Aronne graduated Phi Beta Kappa from Trinity College with a BS in biochemistry and from Johns Hopkins University School of Medicine. He completed his internship and residency at Albert Einstein College of Medicine and the Bronx Municipal Hospital Center, followed by a Henry J. Kaiser Family Foundation Fellowship at New York Hospital-Cornell Medical Center. He is a member of the Alpha Omega Alpha Medical Honor Society.

Dr. Aronne is a former president of the Obesity Society, a fellow of the American College of Physicians, and vice chairman of the board of the American Board of Obesity Medicine. He has authored more than sixty papers and book chapters on obesity and edited the National Institutes of Health *Practical Guide to the Identification, Evaluation, and Treatment of Overweight and Obesity in Adults.* He served as a consultant to the VA Weight Management/Physical Activity Executive Council in the development of the MOVE program, the nation's largest medically based weight control program. Dr. Aronne has won several awards for medical teaching, including the Davidoff Prize from Albert Einstein College of Medicine and the Elliot Hochstein Award from Cornell University.

He lives in Connecticut with his wife, Jane.

# INDEX

\* Recipes can be found in a separate
  index.

**A**

Abdominal fat, 24
  gender and, 23
  types of, 23
Abnormal blood lipids or fats, 13
ACE (angiotensin-converting enzyme)
    inhibitors, 43
Acrp30/apm-1/GBP28, 68
Active, getting, 217–220
Actos, 43–44
Adenosine, caffeine in blocking, 39
Adenovirus 36, 53–55
Adipokines, 61
Adiponectin, 61
Adipose tissue, 60
Adjustable gastric band, xxii, 268–270,
    274
Adrenaline, 223
Agave nectar, 87
Age
  body mass index and, 21
  metabolic, 38
Aging, muscle loss in, xxi–xxii
Agouti gene, 32
AGRP, 68
Air conditioning, 46–47
Akt, 37–38
Alcohol, 107
Al dente cooking, 109
Allegra, 41

Allergies, 40–41
  weight gain and, 41
Alli, 251
Alzheimer's disease, 15
Amaryl, 43, 80
American College of Surgeons Metabolic
    and Bariatric Surgery, 265
American Heart Association on sugar
    intake, 83
American Society for Metabolic and
    Bariatric Surgery, 265
Amino acids, 121
Amygdala, 37
Angina, 12
Angiotensin, 61
Angiotensin-converting enzyme (ACE)
    inhibitors, 43
Angiotensin II, 24
Angiotensin receptor blockers (ARBs),
    43
Animal proteins, 120–121
  casein or milk protein, 121
  egg white protein, 121
  whey protein in, 120–121
Antihistamines, 40–42
Antipsychotics, 45
Antiseizure medications, 44–45
Apidra, 44
Appetite
  ghrelin and, 36–37
  leptin and, 36–37
ARBs (angiotensin receptor blockers),
    43

Aripiprazole (Abilify), 45
Aronne, Jane, ix, 312
Aronne, Lou, ix, 312
Arthritis, obesity and, xiv
Artificial sweeteners, consumption of, 107–108
AspireAssist, 281–282
Asthma, obesity and, xiv, 15
Atacand, 43
Avandia, 43–44
Avapro, 43
Avian virus, 53

**B**

Back pain, reducing lower, 17
Backsliding phenomenon, 4
Bananas and skim milk diet, 9
Banting, William, 8
Belly fat, 15, 24
    losing, 24–25
Benadryl (diphenhydramine), 41
Benicar, 43
Benzphetamine, 254
Beta-blockers, 42–43
Betaine, 33
Bircher-Benner, Maximilian, 8
Blanching, 149
Blood pressure medications, xxii, 42–43
Blood sugar. *See also* Diabetes
    Akt in regulating, 38
    physical activity in lowering, 221–223
Blood thinners, 80
BMI. *See* Body mass index (BMI)
BMIQ, 286, 312
Body, resistance to weight loss, 66–68
Body mass index (BMI), 19–23
    adding medications to weight loss program, 249
    age and, 21

body composition and, 21
calculators of, 19
ethnicity and, 21–22
fat location and, 21
fat tissue and, 61
gender and, 22
genetics in determining, 30
sleep deprivation and, 36
weight ranges for, 20
Body weight set point, 65
BPA (bisphenol A), 49, 50
    avoiding, 50
Brain
    effect of inactivity on, 215–217
    food addiction and, 69–72
    metabolic messaging system in, 63
    vagus nerve and, 69
Bread
    in Change Your Biology Diet, 143–145
    healthy options, 145
    saying no to, 103–105
Breakfast
    in Change Your Biology Diet, 144–145
    having protein for, 102–103
    recipe for, 164–165
    skipping, 106
Breakthrough Dozen, xx, 101, 102–113, 136
Breast cancer
    obesity and, xiv
    soy and, 122
Brillat-Savarin, Jean-Anthelme, 7
Brown fat, 47
    activating, 47, 225
    turning white fat to, 224–225
Brown rice protein, 122
Bupropion (Wellbutrin), 42
B vitamins, 32, 33
Bydureon, 44

Byetta, 44
Byron, Lord, 7
Bystolic, 43

**C**

Cabbage and fruit diet, 9
Caduel, 43
Caffeine in blocking adenosine, 39
Calcium caseinate, 121
Calcium channel blockers, 43
Calories
  avoiding in drinks, 107
  counting, 8
Calories Don't Count Diet, 10
Cameron, Robert, 11
Cancer
  risk of, 14
  starting diet and, 80
Capoten, 43
Carbamazepine, 80
Carbohydrates, 87
  al dente cooking and, 109
  complex, 87, 88–89
  refined, 6
  simple, 87–93, 135
Cardiovascular diseasse, 12
  lowering risk factors for, 16
Casein, 121
Catecholamines, 223, 224
Caveman diet, 11
Celiac disease, 5
Central obesity, 23
Change Your Biology Diet, xx, 135–151
  being active with, 211, 217–220
  breads and grains in, 143–145
  breakfast in, 144–145
  dairy products iin, 141
  dinner in, 147–148
  fats and condiments in, 142
  flexibility of, 285
  free foods in, 151

fruits in, 140
locking in weight loss in, 137–138
lunch in, 147
meal-by-meal guidelines for, 144–151
meat and other sources of protein in, 139
overview of, 97–100
pantry for, 133–134
science behind, xviii, 16, 285
snacks in, 149–150
vegetables in, 138–139
weight control in, 136–137
Change Your Biology Diet Meal Plans, xxi, 152–162
  making it easy, 152–154
  not feeling like cooking, 162
  portion sizes, 155
CHAOS, 59–60
Chicken, recipes for, 189–197
Childhood obesity, xiv, 3, 30
Cholecycstokinin, 68
Cholesterol
  HDL, 13, 95
  LDL, 95
  medications in controlling, xxii
Choline, 33
Cider vinegar and water diet, 7
Cigarette diet, 8
Claritin, 41
Clozapine (Clozarif), 45
Complex carbohydrates, 87, 88–89
Comprehensive Weight Control Center, xiii, 112, 285, 287
Condiments in Change Your Biology Diet, 142
Congestive heart failure, starting diet and, 80
Convenience, 29
Convenience foods, 153
Coreg, 43

Coronary heart disease
  risk of, 16
  starting diet and, 80
Corticotropin-releasing hormone, 67
Cortisol, sleep deprivation and, 37
Cost-effective care, xii
Coumadin, 80
Cozaar, 43
CPAP (continuous positive airway
    pressure) machine, 38
C-reactive protein (CRP), 61
Cymbalta, 42
Cytokines, 24, 41

**D**

Daily log, keeping, 110–111
Dairy products in Change Your Biology
    Diet, 141
Demenia, 15
Depression, obesity and, xiv
Dexamethasone (Decadron and
    Hexadrol), 44
DiaBeta, 43
Diabetes, 13, 38. *See also* Blood sugar
  medications in controlling, xxii,
    43–44
  obesity and, xiv
  reducing risk of, 16
  starting diet and, 80
Diallyl sulphide (DADS), 33
Diet(s)
  bananas and skim milk, 9
  breaking away from the standard
    American (or Western), 83–86
  cabbage and fruit, 9
  calories don't count, 10
  caveman, 11
  cider vinegar and water, 7
  cigarette, 8
  drinking man's, 11
  eating right for your type, 11

fad, xix, 11, 12
grapefruit, 9
hay, 9
high-protein, 81
history of, 7–12, 79
Hollywood, 9
hunter-gatherer, 9
Inuit meat and fad, 9
low-carbohydrate, 7, 8, 81, 110,
    111
low-fat, 81
low-flycemic, 81–82
magic bullet, xix
Mediterranean, 83, 135
methyl-deficient, 33
mondo, 4–7
paleo, 11
raw food, 8, 11
Scarsdake, 11
sleeping beauty, 11
standard American, 83–86
talking with doctor before starting,
    80–83
tapeworm, 8
Weight Watchers, 10
zen macrobiotic, 10
Diethylpropion, 254
Diet industry, earnings in, 4
Dieting, yo-yo, xix, xxii
Dinner in Change Your Biology Diet,
    147–148
Diovan, 43
Dips, recipes for, 165–169
DNA, 32
  viral, 54
DNA methylation, 32
Doctors
  raising awareness in, 286
  seeing your, 112–113
  talking to about medications,
    40

talking with, before starting diet, 80–83
treatment of obesity and, xiv
Dopamine, 68, 71
Douglas, R. Gordon, xiii
Drinking Man's Diet, 11
Drinks, avoiding calories in, 107
Dr. Stoll's Diet Aid, 9

E
Eating
changes in, following surgery, 276–278
of protein at meals, 103
time-restricted, 106
Eating Right for Your Type diet, 11
Economics, weight gain and, 28
Effexor, 42
Eggs, versatility of, 153–154
Egg substitutes, versatility of, 153–154
Egg whites, 121
versatility of, 153–154
Elavil, 42
EndoBarrier, 283
Endocrine disruptors, 48, 49, 121
Epigenetics, xviii, 31–32, 34
Epigenome, 31–32
Epilepsy, starting diet and, 80
Ethnicity, body mass index and, 21–22
Etingin, xiii
Exercise(s)
adding to day, 17
back extension, 231–232, 237–238
benefits of, 109–110
calf raises, 229
classic push-up, 242
curling up, 245
diamond push-up, 243
double crunch, 239–240
dynamic prone plank, 244
elevated calf raise, 234–235

elevated glute bridge, 245
finding time for, 211
full plank, 238–239
getting active and, 217–220
glute bridge, 232–233
increasing intensity in, 220–224, 226
knee plank, 232
lunges, 240–241
one-legged calf raise, 241
push-up from the knees, 235–236
push-ups, 229
seated dumbbell triceps extension, 230–231
seated two-handed dumbbell extension, 236–237
sleep deprivation and, 39
spot, 25
squats, 228–229
static crunch, 233–234
superman, 243–244
turning white fat to brown fat, 224–225
two-step approach to, xxi, 110
wall push-up, 230
wall sit, 234
working muscles in, 225–238
"Exercise snacks," 223
Exforg, 43
Extra-virgin olive oil, 94–97

F
Fad diets, xix
basis of, 12
identifying, 11
Farxiga, 44
Fasts, 11
Fat cells
as endocrine organs, 60–61
function of, xix
producing of leptin, 62–63

Fat cells (*cont.*)
   release of cytokines, 41
   response to sleep deprivation, 37–38
Fats
   in Change Your Biology Diet, 142
   research on, 93–94
   turning white to brown, 224–225
Fattening factors, 27–55
   air conditioning as, 46–47
   BPA (bisphenol A) as, 50
   convenience and, 29
   genes as, 30–34
   labor saving devices as, 29–30
   medications as, 39–46
   obesogens as, 48–50
   organotins-TBT as, 51
   phthalate plasticers as, 52
   phytoestrogens as, 50–51
   sleep deprivation as, 35–39
   social network as, 52–52
"Feed-forward" mechanism, 62
Fiber, 88
Fight-or-flight response, 223
Fish and seafood, recipes for, 198–204
FODMAPS, 6
Folate, 32
Folic acid, 33
Food, avoiding boxed, 106–107
Food addiction, 69–72
   role in obesity, xviii
Food marketing, 29
Food subsidies, 28
Food timing, xx–xxi
Framingham Heart Study, 52
Free foods in Change Your Biology Diet, 151
Friedman, Jeffrey, 62
Frontal cortex, 37
Frozen meals, 162
Fructose, 86–87
Fruits in Change Your Biology Diet, 140

**G**

Galanin, 68
Gallstones, 15, 276
Gastric bypass surgery, xxii, 66
Gastrointestinal disorders, starting diet and, 80
Gender
   abdominal fat and, 23
   body mass index and, 22
   waist circumference and, 22–23
Genes, 30–34
   Agouti, 32
   obesity, 31
Genetics, xviii
Genistein, 50–51
Ghrelin, 36–37, 64, 65–66, 68
GI dynamics endobarrier, 283
Glipizide, 43
Glucagon-like peptide 1, 68
Glucose, 58, 86–87
Glucose intolerance, artificial sweeteners and, 107
Glucotrol, 43, 80
Gluten, 4–5
   research on, 5–6
Gluten-free products, 4, 6
   sales of, 6
Gluten intolerane, 5
Glycemic index, 89–93
Glycemic load, 90–93
   reducing, by changing order of eating, 103
Graham's diet, 7
Graham, Sylvester, 7
Grains in Change Your Biology Diet, 143–145
Grapefruit diet, 9
Ground beef, recipes for, 177–178, 204–205
Guilt, xviii
Gut-brain-gut axis, 68–69

## H

Harrop, George, 9
Hay diet, 9
Hay, William Howard, 9
HbA1c, 13
hCG (human chorionic gonadotropin), 10
HDL (good) cholesterol, 13, 95
Health care problem, weight loss as a, xi–xv
Health threat, obesity as a, 19–26
Heart attack, 12
Heart disease, 38
    medication in controlling, xxii
    obesity and, xiv
Heart failure, 12
Hemp protein, 122
High blood pressure, 12
    controlling, 17
    obesity and, xiv
High-intensity interval training, 220–221
High-intensity resistance training, xxi, 225
High-intensity strength training, xxi
High-protein diet, 81
Histamine, 41
Hollywood diet, 9
Hormones
    visceral fat and, 24
    weight loss and, 56–66
Hot flashes, reducing, 17
HSL (hormone sensitive lipase), 60
Humalog, 44
Human chorionic gonadotropin (hCG), 10
Human Obesity Gene Map, 31
Hummus, 163, 165
Hunger games, winning the, 79–101
Hunter-gatherer diet, 9

Hydrocortisone (Acticort and Cortef), 44
Hypertension, 24, 42–43
    pulmonary, 255–256
    starting diet and, 80
Hypoglycemia, starting diet and, 80
Hypothalamus, 65, 69–70

## I

Illness. See also specific illnesses
    relationship between obesity and, xiii
IMO, 123
Inactivity, effect of, on brain and microbiome, 215–217
Inderal, 43
Infertility, 14
    obesity and, xiv
Inflammatory substances, reducing, 16
InForm Fitness, xxi, 225
Insulin, 37, 57, 79
Insulin resistance, 13, 17, 50, 57–60
    artificial sweeteners and, 107
    blood sugar and, 221
    factors contributing, 60
Intensity, increasing, in exercise, 220–224
Interleukin-6, 24
Interleukins, 61
Interval aerobics training, 285
Interval training, high-intensity, 220–221
Intragastric balloons, xxii, 280–281
Inuit meat and fad diet, 9
Invokana, 44
Irisin, 225
Isoflavones, 50, 122

## J

Jacobs, Jonathan, xiii
Jardiance, 44
Jenkins, David, 89

Juice cleanses, 11
Juice fasts, 4
Junk food, sleep deprivation and, 37

**K**
Kaplan, Lee, xiii
Kidney disease, starting diet and, 80
Kidney failure, 12

**L**
Labor saving devices, 29–30
Lantus, 44
Laparoscopic sleeve gastrectomy, xxii,
    265–268, 274
LDL (bad) cholesterol, 13, 95
Leibel, Rudy, 62
Leptin, 61, 62–64, 67, 69
    appetite and, 36–37
Leptin resistance, 61–65, 79
Letterman, Dave, ix
Lettuce wraps, 153
Levimir, 44
Lifestyle changes, 113
Lifestyle counseling, 282
Lifestyle movement, xxi
Liquids, non-caloric, 100, 107
Liraglutide (Saxanda), 258–259
Lithium, 45, 81
Liver disease, obesity and, xiv
Lopressor, 43
Lorcaserin (Belviq), 255–256
Lotensin, 43
Lotrel, 43
Low-carbohydrate diet, 7, 8, 81, 110,
    111
Low-fat diet, 81
Low-glycemic diet, 81–82
Lunch, in Change Your Biology Diet,
    147
Lurasidone (Latuda), 45
Lyrica, 45

**M**
Magic bullet diets, xix
MAO inhibitors, 81
MCH, 68
Meal replacements
    in jump-starting weight loss,
        114–116
    protein bars as, 114–115
    protein dense, 116
    protein shakes as, 114–115
    shakes as, 125
Meats and other proteins, in Change
    Your Biology Diet, 139
Medications, xxii, 113, 249–262
    antidepressants, 42
    antihistamines, 40–42
    antipsychotics and mood disorder,
        45
    antiseizure, 44–45
    blood pressure, xxii, 42–43
    cholesterol, xxii
    diabetes, xxii, 43–44
    with fattening side effects, 39–46
    heart disease, xxii
    Liraglutide (Saxanda), 258–259
    Lorcaserin (Belviq), 255–256
    Metformin (Glucoghage), 261–262
    obesity treatment gap and, 250–255
    oral corticosteroids, 44
    Phentermine, 260
    Phentermine/Topiramate (Qsymia),
        257–259
    selective serotonin reuptake inhibitors
        (SSRIs), 42
    talking with doctor about, 40
Mediterranean diet, 83, 135
a-Melanocyte-stimulating hromone,
    67
Melatonin, 42
Menopause, 17, 24
Metabolic age, 38

Metabolic syndrome, 14, 21, 50, 60, 116
  brown fat and, 224
  diagnosis of, 14
Metabolism, reving up, 285
Metformin (Glucoghage), 44, 261–262
Methionine, 33
Methyl-donating nutrients, 32–33
Methyl groups, 32
Methylprednisolone (Medrol), 44
Microbiome, 72–75, 79
  effect of inactivity on, 215–217
Middle-age spread, 24
Mondo diet, 4–7
Monopril, 43
Monosaccharides, 86
Mood disorders, starting diet and, 81
Mood stabilizers, 45
Movement, adding in weight loss, xxi
Multigrain products, 143
Muscle exhaustion, 227
Muscle loss, in aging, xxi–xxii
Muscle mass, building, xxi
Muscles
  memory in, 228
  working, 225–238
Muscle tissue, 109

N
NEAT (non-exercise activity thermogenesis), 215
Neuromedin, 68
Neurontin, 45
Neuropeptide Y, 68
New York Hospital-Cornell Medical Center
  Center for Special Studies at, xiii
  Comprehensive Weight Control Center at, xiii, 28, 112, 285
  Woman's Health Center at, xiii
Nidetch, Jean, 10

Norepinephrine, 68, 223, 254
Norvasc, 43
Novalog, 44

O
Obesity
  asthma and, xiv, 15
  BMI in determining, 263
  central, 23
  childhood, xiv, 3, 30
  complications of, 12–16
  death rates associated with severe, 263
  food addiction in, xviii
  frustrations of, 3–4
  global estimates of, xiii
  as health threat, 19–26
  link between asthma and, 15
  as medical problem, xxii–xxiii
  as pandemic, xiii
  relationship between illness and, xiii
  social network and, 52
  as viral, 53–55
Obesity genes, 31
Obesity-related illnesses, xiv
  health care costs of, xiv
Obesity treatment gap, 250–255
Obesogenic environment, 31
Obesogens, 48–50
Obsawa, George, 10
Off-label prescribing, 260
Olanzapine (Zyprexa), 45
Oleic acid, 95
Olive oil, 94–97
  extra virgin, 94–97
  pure, 95
  refined or "light," 95
  virgin, 95
Omega-3 fatty acids, 65
Oral corticosteroids, 44

Orbera intragastric balloons, xxii, 280–281

Orexin/Hypocretin, 68

Organotins, 50, 51

   avoiding, 51

Orli, xiii

Orlistat, 251

Ornish, Dean's, Low-Fat Diet, 11

Osteoarthritiis, 15, 17

Overweight children, increase in numbers of, 30

**P**

Paleo diet, 11

Paltrow, Gwyneth, 10

Pamelor, 42

Pancreatitis, obesity and, xiv

Pantry, for the Change Your Biology Diet, 133–134

Pea protein, 122

Peptide-1 (GLP1), 74

Peptide YY (PYY), 74

Perilipin, 68

Peters, Lulu Hunt, 8

Phendinetrazine, 254

Phenobarbital, 80

Phentermine, 254, 260

Phentermine/Topiramate (Qsymia), 257–259

Phenytoin, 80

Phthalates, 50, 52

   avoiding, 552

Physicians. See Doctors

The Physiology of Taste (Brillat-Savarin), 7

Phytoestrogens, 50–51, 122

   avoiding, 51

Phytonutrients, 95

Plaque, 12

Plateaus, breaking through, 211

Polycystic ovary syndrome, 14

Portion control, 100–101

   importance of, xx–xxi

   protein shakes in, 114

   quick reference for, 155

Post-prandial glucose response, 104

Post-surgery, expectations, 276

Pounds and Inches (Simeons), 10

Power of 10 (Zickerman), xxi, 225

Prebiotics, 74

Prediabetes, 13

   insulin resistance and, 57

   Metformin (Glucoghage) in, 261

Prednisone (Deltasone and Sterapred), 44

Pritikin Program, 11

Processed foods, 83

   as addictive, xviii–xiv, 85, 106

Propionate, 74

Protein, 102

   animal, 120–121

   for breakfast, 102–103

   eating first at meals, 103

   vegetable, 121–125

Protein bars, 114–115

   checking labels of, 123

   recommended, 124

Protein blends, 121

Protein powders, 120, 125

Protein shakes, xx, 114–115, 116–120

   checking labels of, 123

   recipes for, 126–132

   recommended, 124

   turning into treats, 125–133

Prozac, 42

Pulmonary hypertension, 255–256

**Q**

Quest bars, 123

Quetiapine (Seroquel), 45

Quick Start Change Your Biology Diet, xx, 114–134

animal proteins in, 120–121
flexibility of, 285
levels in, 116–119
meal replacements in, 114–116
pantry for, 133–134
protein bars in, 114–115, 125
protein powders and, 120
protein shakes in, 114–115, 116–119, 124, 125–133, 126–132
vegetable proteins in, 121–125

**R**

Raw food diet, 8, 11
Refined carbohydrates, 6
Remeron, 42
Remote controls, 29–30
Re Muscle Health bars, 123
Re Muscle Health shakes, 123
Reproductive abnormalities, 14
ReShape intragastric balloons, xxii, 280–281
Resistance training, xxi–xxii, 110, 225–226
high-intensity, xxi
Resistin, 61
Resveratrol, 33
Risperidone (Risperdal), 45
Roux-en-y gastric bypass, 271–273, 275

**S**

Salad dressings, recipes for, 169–174
Salads, 153
Sarcopenia, 109
Sauces, recipes for, 184–189
Scarsdale Diet, 11
Science, behind Change Your Biology Diet, xviii, 16, 285
Seizure disorders, starting diet and, 80
Selective serotonin reuptake inhibitors (SSRIs), 42
Serotonin, 68, 97, 255

Serotonin reuptake inhibitors (SSRIs), 256
Sexual dysfunction, 14
obesity and, xiv
SGLT-2 inhibitors, 44
Shame, xviii
Sides, recipes for, 205–210
Simeons, A. T., 10
Simple carbohydrates, 87–93, 135
Simple sugars, 86–87
Sitting, negative consequences of, 212–215
Sleep apnea, 15, 17, 38
Sleep deprivation, 35–39
Sleeping Beauty Diet, 11
Sleeve gastrectomy, xxii
Slimming soaps, 9
SMAM-1, 53
Snacks, 105–106
in Change Your Biology Diet, 149–150
Social network, 52–53
Somatostatin, 68
Soups, recipes for, 174–183
Soy protein, 121–122
Spot exercise, 25
Spreads, recipes for, 165–169
SSRIs (selective serotonin reuptake inhibitors), 42
Standard American diet (SAD), breaking away from, 83–86
Standing, benefits of, 214–215
Steamer basket, 153
Stefansson, Vilhalmur, 9
Stir fry, 153, 163
building a, 183–184
Strength training, 110, 212
high-intensity, xxi
Stroke, 12
obesity and, xiv
Subcutaneous fat, 23

Sucrose, 83, 86–87
Sugar, 83
    consumption of, 83
    names for, 84–85
    simple, 86–87
Sulforaphane, 33
Surgery
    adjustable gastric band, xxii,
        268–270, 274
    AspireAssist, 281–282
    being candidate for, 264
    changes in earting following,
        276–278
    comparison of, 273–276
    EndoBarrier, 283
    expectations following, 276
    GI dynamics endobarrier, 283
    intragastric balloons, xxii, 280–281
    laparoscopic sleeve gastrectomy, xxii,
        265–268, 274
    reality versus expectations, 278–279
    roux-en-y gastric bypass, xxii, 66,
        271–273, 275
    vBloc vagal nerve stimulator, xxii,
        69, 279–280
Symlin, 44
Sympathetic nervous system, effect of
    strenuous exercise on, 223

T

Taller, Herman, 10
Tapeworm diet, 8
    side effects of, 8
Target weight, 16
TBT (tributyltin), 51
Tegretol, 45
Telomeres, 214
Temperature-controlled environment,
    46–47
Tenormin, 43
Thermoneutral zone (TNZ), 47
Thermoregulation, 47

Thiazolidinediones, 43–44
Thryotropin-releasing hormone, 68
Thyroid hormone, 56–57
Time-restricted eating, 106
TNF-a (tumor necrosis factor alpha),
    24, 61
Topamax, 45
Treats, turning protein shakes into,
    125–133
Tricyclic antidepressants, 42
Triglycerides, 59
Trulicity, 44
Tumor necrosis factor alpha (TNF-a),
    24, 61
Turkey, recipe for, 197–198
2C receptors, 255
Two-step approach to exercise, 110

U

United Fruit Company, 9
Urocortin, 68

V

Vagus nerve, 68–69, 79
    vBloc Maestro System in targeting,
        279–280
Valproic acid (Depakote and Depakene),
    44
Vasotec, 43
vBloc Maestro system, 279–280
vBloc vagal nerve stimulator, xxii,
    69, 279–280
Vegetable proteins, 121–125
    brown rice protein, 122
    hemp protein, 122
    pea protein, 122
    soy protein, 121–122
Vegetables
    in Change Your Biology Diet,
        138–139
    eating first at meals, 103
    roasted, 153

Victoza, 44
Viral DNA, 52
Visceral fat, 23, 24, 26, 122
  breakdown of, 24
  ghrelin in storage of, 66
  losing, 24–25
Vitamin B6, 33
Vitamin B12, 32, 33

**W**

Waist circumference, 19, 22–23
Waist-to-height ratio, 25–26
Weighing, regular, 112
Weight-centric approach, 18–19
Weight gain
  dynamics of, xviii
  economics and, 28
  fat cell metabolism and, 59
  fattening factors in, 27–55
  rate of, xxii
  science behind, xviii
Weight loss
  adding movement in, xxi
  benefits of, 286
  body resistance to, 66–68
  Breakthrough Dozen and, xx, 101,
    102–113
  in Change Your Biology Diet,
    136–137
  changing the way you eat in, xxi
  difficulty of, xi
  fat cells and, 60–61
  food addiction and, 69–70
  ghrelin and, 65–66
  gut-brain-gut axis and, 68–69
  as health care problem, xi–xv
  hormones and, 56–66
  insulin resistance and, 57–60
  jump-starting, 285
  leptin resistance and, 61–65
  locking in, in Change Your Biology
    Diet, 137–138

  meal replacements in jump-starting,
    114–116
  medications for, xxii, 249–262
  microbiome and, 72–75
  as problem, 3–4
  speed of, 116
  turning around, 16–19
  willpower in, xi–xii, xiii
Weight loss resistance, xii
  biology of, xviii
Weight management program, need for
    realistic goals in, 11
Weight Watchers, 10
Weill Cornell Medical College, xi, xii,
    xiii
  Comprehensive Weight Control
    Center at, xiii, 112, 285, 287
Wheelies, 30
Whey concentrate, 120–121
Whey isolate, 121
Whey protein, 120–121
White fat, 47
  turning to brown fat, 224–225
Willpower, in weight loss, xi–xii, xiii

**X**

Xenical, 251

**Y**

Yo-yo dieting, xix, xxii

**Z**

Zen Buddhism, 10
Zen Macrobiotic Diet, 10
Zhang, Yiying, 62
Zickerman, Adam, xxi, 110, 212,
    225
Ziprasidone (Geodon), 45
Zoloft, 42
The Zone, 11
Zonegran, 45
Zyrtec, 41

# RECIPE INDEX

**B**

Breakfast
    Cheese and Veggie "Cupcake"
        Omelets, 164–165

**C**

Chicken
    Basic Chicken Soup from Scratch,
        175
    Broiled Country Mustard Chicken,
        196–197
    Chicken and Spinach Soup with Pesto,
        176–177
    Chicken Breast with Asparagus and
        Carrots in a Parchment Packet,
        191–192
    Pepper Chicken Casserole, 195
    Poached Chicken and Vegetables,
        190–191
    Quick Roast Lemon Chicken,
        189–190
    Tandoori Chicken, 195–196
    Vinegar Chicken, 194
    White Bean, Escarole, and Chicken
        Sausage Soup, 180–181

**F**

Fish and Seafood, 198–205
    Broiled Flounder with Ginger-Lime
        Sauce, 203–204
    Broiled Tilapia with Tangy Sauce, 200
    Parchment-Baked Halibut, 202–203
    Red Snapper Creole, 198–199

    Salmon with Red Pesto, 199–200
    Sautéed Bass with Shiitake Mushroom
        Sauce, 201–202
    Seared Scallops with Cherry Tomatoes
        and Fennel, 201
    Shrimp and Scallop Stew, 182–183

**G**

Ground beef
    Blue Plate Special Meat Loaf,
        204–205
    Sweet-and-Sour Beef Soup, 177–178

**P**

Protein Shakes
    An Apple a Day . . . , 128
    Berry Medley, 129
    Black and Blue, 128
    Cherries in the Snow, 130
    Chocolate-Covered Cherries, 130
    Cinnamon Roll, 130–131
    Coconut Almond Treat, 131
    A Fine Use for Leftover Coffee, 126
    Harvest Pumpkin Pie, 132
    Kiwi and Blueberry Shake, 130
    Mocha Mint, 126–127
    Mocha Pick Me Up, 126
    Old-Fashioned Lemon Square Shake,
        131–132
    Peaches and Cream, 127
    Peachy Keen, 131
    Pina Colada, 132
    Red Velvet, 132

Refreshing Melon Shake, 128–129
Sinfully Chocolate, 127
Strawberries Dipped in Chocolate, 127–128
Thick Raspberry Chocolate Shake, 129

**S**

Salad Dressings, 169–174
Champagne Vinaigrette, 169–170
Creamy Curry Dressing, 174
Creamy Dill Ranch, 173–174
Greek Island Dressing, 172
Green Goddess Dressing, 173
Herbed Cucumber Vinaigrette, 171
Low-Calorie Creamy Caesar, 171–172
Simple Asian Vinaigrette, 170–171
Zesty Lemon-Mint Vinaigrette, 170
Sauces, 184–189
Butterless White Wine Sauce, 185
Cherry Tomato Sauce, 188–189
Chimichurri Sauce, 186
Fresh Vegetable Sauce, 187–188
Garlicky Chickpea Sauce, 185–186
Herbed Mustard Sauce, 188
Sides
Baked Zucchini, 209–210
Can't Believe It's Not Mashed Potatoes, 206–207
Hot Lentil Salad, 208–209
Roasted Vegetables, 205–206

Vegetable Quinoa, 207–208
Snacks
Cheese and Veggie "Cupcake" Omelets, 164–165
Soups
Basic Chicken Soup from Scratch, 175
Black Bean Soup, 181–182
Broccoli Soup, 178
Chicken and Spinach Soup with Pesto, 176–177
EZ Vegetable Soup, 179
Hearty Vegetable Soup, 179–180
Shrimp and Scallop Stew, 182–183
Sweet-and-Sour Beef Soup, 177–178
White Bean, Escarole, and Chicken Sausage Soup, 180–181
Spreads and Dips, 165–169
Avocado Yogurt Dip with a Kick, 165
Cool Dip, 166–167
Mediterranean Bean Dip, 166
Nutty Edamame Spread, 167
Olive-Mustard Tapenade, 168–169
Sun-Dried Tomato and White Bean Dip, 168

**T**

Turkey
Turkey Piccata, 197–198